Workplace Learning in Health and Social Care

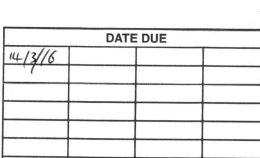

Workplace Learning in Health and Social Care

A Student's Guide

Edited by Carolyn Jackson and Claire Thurgate

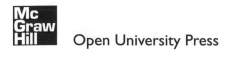

Open University Press

Open University Press
McGraw-Hill Education
McGraw-Hill House
Shoppenhangers Road
Maidenhead
Berkshire
England
SL6 2QL

email: enquiries@openup.co.uk
world wide web: www.openup.co.uk

and Two Penn Plaza, New York, NY 10121-2289, USA

First published 2011

A catalogue record of this book is available from the British Library

ISBN-13: 978-0-33-523750-0 (pb) 978-0-33-523749-4 (hb)

Library of Congress Cataloging-in-Publication Data
CIP data applied for

Typeset by RefineCatch Limited, Bungay, Suffolk
Printed in the UK by Bell and Bain Ltd, Glasgow.

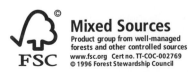

Mixed Sources
Product group from well-managed
forests and other controlled sources
www.fsc.org Cert no. TT-COC-002769
© 1996 Forest Stewardship Council

FSC

The *McGraw-Hill* Companies

Contents

**Part 1   Introducing work based learning – how does learning
happen in the workplace?**

Part 3   The benefits and challenges of learning in the workplace and future career development planning

9 Career planning for the future – where to from here?   **112**
Carolyn Jackson

Figures

Tables

List of contributors

Jane Abbott MSc, BA (Hons), Cert Ed, CM, RN. Jane is Hospital Director at the Benenden Hospital Trust. During her career Jane has been Director of Nursing at the Benenden Hospital as well as holding senior management positions within the NHS. Jane has always had an interest in the educational development of her staff and was for a period of time clinical education lead in the Renal Unit at St George's Hospital, London, where she had a special interest in the education of healthcare support workers.

Tom Aird MA History of Education, PG Dip Clinical Neuroscience, BA (Hons) Nurse Education, RNT, RGN. Tom is Principal Lecturer in the Faculty of Health and Social Care at London South Bank University. After qualifying as a Registered Nurse from the Southern General Hospital in Glasgow in 1979, Tom has worked in a variety of intensive care and neurosurgical units, both in the UK and the USA. Since starting in education in 1989 his role has undergone significant changes which have helped him meet the changing demands of the health and social care sector. The biggest change took place in 2001 when he took on a strategic role to develop and implement a work based learning framework for the post-qualifying students in addition to advising on work based learning elements of the Foundation Degrees being developed. The role currently includes **APEL** and Distance Learning. Consequently the role has an emphasis on educational programmes and activities outside the traditional classroom. Being involved with work based learning enables Tom to discuss individual development needs with key stakeholders addressing specific organizational needs.

Jayne Crow MSc, BA (Hons), RGN, Dip N (Lond), Cert. Ed. Jayne is a Senior Lecturer at Anglia Ruskin University and has many years experience teaching both Health and Social Work students on a wide range of pre- and post-qualifying courses from Foundation Degree to postgraduate awards. She came to Higher Education from a career in adult nursing and has a specific interest in health psychology, interprofessional learning, collaborative working and Action Research.

Peter Ellis MA, MSc, BSc (Hons), PGCE, PGCM, RN. Peter is a Senior Lecturer in the Department of Nursing and Applied Clinical Studies at Canterbury Christ Church University. Peter leads on the delivery of Leadership and Management modules within the department and is involved in collaborative leadership teaching across the university. Peter has also taught evidence-based practice on the Foundation Degree. Prior to joining Canterbury Christ Church University, Peter was Senior Nurse for renal outpatients and Research Projects Manager in the Renal Unit at King's College Hospital, London.

Carolyn Jackson MSc, PGDEd, RNT, Dip (Coaching and Mentoring), BA, RGN. Carolyn is Head of Department for Nursing and Applied Clinical Studies in the Faculty of Health and Social Care at Canterbury Christ Church University. She has been working in higher education in the UK, Europe and Australasia since 1991 and prior to that held a number of senior nursing posts in the field of critical care nursing. Carolyn's interests are in the development of effective workplace cultures through education, practice development and research. She has led a number of key **strategic** curriculum developments at Foundation Degree to PhD level that have directly influenced workforce developments and the creation of new roles at specialist and advanced practice level. Currently she is involved in projects and collaborations aimed at enhancing the quality of health professional education at the European level and nationally in the modernizing of future nursing, midwifery and allied health professional careers.

Mary Northrop MSc Medical Sociology, BA (Hons) Combined Studies Sociology and Literature, Dip HE Nursing, RMN, RGN, RNT, PGCEA. Mary is currently a Senior Lecturer and Pathway leader for a Foundation Degree in Healthcare at Anglia Ruskin University. She has been involved with teaching both pre- and post-registration nurses and developing and delivering pre-professional pathways. She completed a Master's in Medical Sociology at Royal Holloway and prior to that a combined degree in Sociology and Literature at Kingston University. She has worked as a nurse in both adult and mental health settings and is a Registered Nurse Tutor. Her professional interests include sociology of risk, public health and development of new roles in the NHS.

Helen O'Keefe RGN, BSc (Hons) Professional Practice, MSc Nursing Research and Practice Development. Helen is Associate Director of Nursing for Workforce Development, Education and Training at East Kent Hospitals University NHS Foundation Trust. After training as a general nurse at St Bartholomew's Hospital School of Nursing in the early 1980s, Helen gained experience in a variety of clinical specialties before spending most of her clinical career in intensive care nursing. She has worked in higher education, practice development, and spent four years as a nurse consultant in critical care before moving to East Kent. Helen's current role focuses on workforce development and ensuring practitioners are prepared with the appropriate skills, knowledge and experience in order to deliver improved care to patients. She is passionate about the value of work based learning, ensuring that programmes remain responsive to service need and are competency-based. She works closely with university colleagues in developing role-focused accredited work based learning programmes.

Claire Thurgate MA, PGCLT, BSc (Hons), Dip HE, RSCN, RGN. Claire is currently Programme Director for Foundation Degrees in the Faculty of Health and Social Care at Canterbury Christ Church University. Her research interests are in supporting the Associate Practitioner role. She is committed to working with local employers in the health and social care sector to ensure that the future workforce is prepared for the delivery of healthcare 2020. She has presented papers related to collaborative working in Foundation Degrees, students' experiences of transition into higher education and working with employers to assess Foundation Degrees.

Barbara Workman DProf, MSc, BSc (Hons), RN, RNT, RCNT, FHEA. Barbara is Director for the Centre of Excellence in Work Based Learning at Middlesex University. She has a background of nursing and teaching with expertise and research interests in accreditation of organizational and individual learning, and facilitation of work based learning across all higher education levels. She is committed to sharing, spreading and facilitating good practice in work based learning across a range of higher education activities and is a University Teaching Fellow. She has published on learning from work, clinical skills and negotiated work based learning.

Foreword

Jan Dewing

Head of Person-Centred Research and Practice Development, East Sussex Community Trust

Learning in and from everyday life, including from our work, makes a huge contribution to our personal well-being and ultimately to our ability to thrive and flourish as people in the world. As people, we are presented with a constant neverending source of learning opportunities. When working with people who are ill or vulnerable in some way, those of us in caring and therapeutic roles have a responsibility to ensure that we not only provide care that is as safe as possible (including evidence-informed interventions) but care that is offered in the way that adds to the dignity and self-worth of each person. To do this means staying fresh and re-energized, even in a job that is physically and/or emotionally hard labour a lot of the time. Learning from everyday activity and routines is vital, even for the most experienced healthcare worker. Consequently, healthcare workers in all roles need to learn, and to learn in a number of ways.

There is a relationship between the workplace as a centre of learning, personal and team effectiveness and improved patient care and experience. The workplace that has a multi-faceted learning culture values curiosity, **creativity**, and exploration, and encourages contributions by everyone. It also offers nurturing and can sustain workers' engagement in their work (i.e. their patients). This is a healthy workplace that promotes well-being and thriving in workers and patients. As healthcare seeks to provide safer patient care alongside improved experiences of care, the organization that values and promotes a learning culture for all and seeks out better ways of working for staff, in conjunction with its local communities, improves its capabilities and its reputation. Healthcare organizations can improve quality and safety by enhancing the capability for learning within workplaces and teams – although there must be a recognition that this is far more extensive than simply 'training' workers.

Central to this achieving of the desired outcomes is learning in the workplace; all those vastly differing care settings across an organization should form the heart of learning. About ten years ago, Boud and Garrick described learning at work as one of the most exciting areas of development in the fields of education – and management. This is arguably still a development to reach its potential. However, being committed to learning in and from work requires resources. Some of those resources are internal to each of us, such as curiosity and motivation, while some can be found in the workplace in other colleagues and in the formal learning opportunities that are provided. A core resource is knowing how to go about learning and how to organize learning as a self-directed learner so it becomes a healthy activity rather than something associated with mandatory training or time out. The topic and themes in this book will help healthcare workers become energized, reflective learners who are better placed to provide effective person-centred care.

If you are undertaking a Foundation Degree or another course to support your career progression, there are a wide range of activities in this book to help you make the most of learning opportunities in the workplace. It will help you to explore the career plans and choices you have made to date and show you how to develop your knowledge and skills in a targeted way for the future to make the most of career development opportunities open to you. Most importantly, this book emphasizes the importance of developing good working relationships with people who are concerned for your well-being and want you to thrive, including workplace managers, colleagues and mentors, and course tutors, all of whom can help you make the most of learning opportunities in the workplace.

Preface

Work based learning (WBL) has become increasingly important over the past decade as the UK government strives to create a more flexible cost-effective workforce who learn at work rather than in the traditional classroom setting. There is an increasing emphasis on helping more people, previously excluded from traditional forms of university education, to learn and develop within the workplace. Many employers are supporting programmes of study such as Foundation Degrees (FD) which focus on the knowledge and skills required to undertake new roles such as Assistant/ Associate Practitioners.

WBL differs from the more traditional forms of learning as learning is directly linked to your role in the workplace. Seagraves et al. (1996) identify three strands to work based learning: learning at work, learning for work and learning through work. *Learning at work* involves attending learning events that help you to be effective in undertaking your daily role such as in-house study days. *Learning for work* could involve the development of specific knowledge and skills through a workplace competency tool, or your annual appraisal or Knowledge and Skills Framework or National Occupational Standards. *Learning through* work involves making sense of new knowledge and applying this to the workplace so that you can enhance the quality of the care you provide to your patients or clients.

This book demonstrates how you can learn in the middle of practice and how you can relate theory to practice to transform your understanding of ways in which you work and learn as individuals, and collectively with colleagues in multi-disciplinary teams. It serves as a practical guide for people who are undertaking a Foundation Degree or other work based learning courses to help gain a deeper understanding of the concept of learning at and for work. It aims to support your development through a range of practical strategies and exercises that will strengthen your capacity to learn at work and to reflect on your own personal and professional development goals. The intention is to encourage you to maximize opportunities for continual personal growth at an individual level, at a team level and potentially in turn at an organizational level. It will share the experiences of students, employers and facilitators of learning to develop your understanding of how to capitalize on lifelong learning opportunities to enhance your current and future career development.

Structure of the book

The book is divided into three Parts. Part 1 introduces you to the concept of WBL and explores how learning happens in the workplace. It is designed to help you understand the theoretical underpinnings of WBL, its links to lifelong learning, and your own individual personal development. The learning outcomes for Part 1 are that you should be able to do the following:

- demonstrate an understanding of the concept of work based learning;

- identify different forms of learning in the workplace;

- understand the link between work based learning and lifelong learning to promote personal professional career development.

In Chapter 1, Tom Aird introduces you to the concept of WBL from a theoretical perspective and its links with lifelong learning. He explores why WBL is important and what role it plays in workforce and individual professional development. In Chapter 2, Carolyn Jackson explores the impact that workplace culture has on opportunities for you to learn in the workplace. It explores different forms of learning and discusses the roles that the organization, the multi-disciplinary team, and individual practitioners play in creating a suitable **learning environment** to promote effective workplace learning. It explores the importance of collaborative partnership working in promoting learning in the workplace. In Chapter 3, Barbara Workman helps you to understand your own personal **learning styles** and preferences, and identifies how different forms of learning may be evidenced in the workplace. She discusses how to maximize support for your own personal learning in the workplace.

Part 2 of the book explores how you might demonstrate evidence of learning in the workplace. It uses a range of activities and exercises to let you identify opportunities to learn at work. It will enhance your own self-awareness of your development needs and how to evidence these effectively. It further develops your awareness of the importance of developing key relationships with employers and members of your multi-disciplinary team in order to promote collaboration in WBL. The overall learning outcomes for Part 2 are that you should be able to do the following:

- use a range of tools and methods of reflection and evaluation to help you make the most of your ongoing learning and development;

- write a learning contract and action plan to support workplace development;

- identify which sources of support are available to you in the workplace to help you learn;

- write a Personal Development Plan and use this to think about your future role development;

- explore ways in which you might link your own learning to the Knowledge Skills Framework and Skills for Health competencies to plan for future career development and learning.

In Chapter 4, Mary Northrop introduces the concept of reflection on and in practice to promote learning at work. She guides you through theories and practical strategies to help you reflect on practice, understand the role that reflection plays in demonstrating evidence of learning in the workplace and explore different models of reflection that promote WBL. In Chapter 5, Jayne Crow shows you how to apply reflective theory to practice to promote work based learning, to further develop your reflection skills to promote lifelong learning and understand the range of evidence that can be presented when demonstrating reflection on and in action in the workplace. She presents a range of practical tools and scenarios that will deepen your understanding of how to make the most of reflection. In Chapter 6, Barbara Workman gives practical advice regarding the management of WBL through the use of learning contracts and action plans. She discusses how to use a **mentor** to support your learning in the workplace. In Chapter 7, Claire Thurgate discusses the importance of developing an effective Personal Development Plan (PDP) to help you demonstrate learning in the workplace. She explores the role of personal development planning in formulating goals for WBL and future career development. She offers a range of useful hints and tips to allow you to identify your development needs and goals for the future and to understand how to evidence and evaluate this effectively. She also explores the importance of the relationship with service colleagues and facilitators of WBL who promote the development of PDP in partnership with you.

Part 3 of the book explores how employers engage with WBL, outlining the benefits and challenges for your workplace organization and for you as a learner. Contributions include health service managers and Foundation Degree graduate students' experiences. The intention is to promote awareness of the challenges of learning at work and in achieving a balance between providing a service and providing a sound learning environment from an employer's perspective. We explore how work based learning is helping to underpin workforce development, emergent new roles and scopes of practice and end by exploring further opportunities for you to create a defined career plan for the future. The overall learning outcomes for Part 3 are that you should be able to do the following:

- understand the potential benefits of WBL for your employer;

- identify the barriers to WBL in the workplace and how these might be overcome;

- understand how to maximize support from your workplace managers and colleagues when planning to undertake WBL;

- understand some of the benefits and challenges of undertaking Foundation Degrees or other WBL programmes in relation to career enhancement;

- identify your own career pathway and map out your future plans for development.

In Chapter 8, Peter Ellis, Jane Abbott and Helen O'Keefe explore the benefits and barriers to your employer's engagement with programmes of WBL. They discuss how WBL can develop the individual, the service and the organization and how barriers to effective learning can be overcome. They emphasize the importance of collaborative working in promoting effective WBL and explore ways in which you can make the most of gaining support from the workplace. Students share their experiences of undertaking Foundation Degree study and how this has prepared them to undertake new roles within the health and social care sector. In Chapter 9, Carolyn Jackson provides a practical guide to answer the question 'Where to from here?' It contains evaluative exercises that enable you to develop a coherent career action plan that will act as a guide for your future lifelong learning and career development.

The final chapter of the book is a glossary which presents definitions of the key terms used in this book. The glossary words are shown in bold on their first occurrence.

The book provides quotes and tips from Simon who is a first year student on a Foundation Degree, and Fatima who has completed her Foundation Degree, plus practical guidelines and Time Out activities to let you monitor your own learning and development. It will enable you to question and reflect on your own practice, and develop new insights into your strengths and areas that you need to work on. Many of the exercises will be useful if you are undertaking a course such as a Foundation Degree because they allow you to develop the skills you require to write personal development plans, learning contracts, reflective diaries, and a professional portfolio. If you are not yet undertaking a course but hope to do so in the near future, the activities and exercises will give you detailed insight into your learning styles and preferences, and which aspects of your career you hope to develop and focus on in the future. This in turn will prepare you for the challenges of studying a course or programme at university. We hope you will find the book useful and informative and enjoy reading it as much as we have enjoyed writing it.

Reference

Seagraves, L., Osbourne, M., Neal, P., Dockrell, R., Hartshorn, C. and Boyd, A. (1996) *Learning in Smaller Companies, (LISC) Final Report.* Stirling: University of Sterling, Educational Policy and Development.

Acknowledgements

We would like to extend our heartfelt thanks to the contributors of this book who have worked tirelessly to produce what we all hope are useful and well-read chapters. We have really enjoyed working with academic colleagues Tom Aird, Jayne Crowe, Mary Northrop, Barbara Workman, Peter Ellis, Jane Abbott, Helen O'Keefe; our past students Debbie Beatty, Mark Head, Lynda Stroud and Elaine Dunbar; and workplace mentors Helen Hatter and Janet Pepper who have supported Foundation Degree students in practice. We look forward to future collaborations with you all. We have learned much from each other on this journey together and thank you for your commitment and dedication to meeting on a regular basis.

Our thanks also to Professor Jan Dewing for her Foreword and for inspiring so many practitioners with the passion to develop their workplace cultures and practices. We would also like to recognize the support from Rachel Crookes at the publishing house for her prompt and honest feedback and communication which have helped to shape our thinking.

Carolyn would like to extend her thanks in particular to her partner Noel for his undaunting support and understanding of the need to spend endless evenings and weekends locked in the study. Claire's gratitude goes to Clive, Ben and Will for their patience and humour and to all the Foundation Degree students whom she has worked with for giving her the inspiration to undertake this project.

The publishers would like to thank the copyright holders of the following material for permission to reproduce material in this book:

Allin, L. and Turnock, C. (2007) *Reflection on and in the Workplace.* Reflection Students.
Driscoll, J. (ed.) (2007) *Practising Clinical Supervision: A Reflective Approach for Healthcare Professionals* (2nd edn). Edinburgh: Baillière Tindall.
Honey, P. and Mumford, A. (2006) *The Learning Styles Questionnaire 80-item Version.* Maidenhead: Peter Honey Publications.

Every effort has been made to trace and acknowledge ownership of copyright and to clear permission for material reproduced in this book. The publishers will be pleased to make suitable arrangements to clear permission with any copyright holders whom it has not been possible to contact.

Abbreviations

CV	curriculum vitae
DH	Department of Health
FD	Foundation Degree
HSC	Health and Social Care
KSF	Knowledge and Skills Framework
LC	Learning Contract
LLL	lifelong learning
NHS	National Health Service
NOS	National Occupational Standards
NQF	National Qualifications Framework
PDP	Personal Development Plan
QAA	Quality Assurance Agency
SMART	Specific, Measurable, Achievable, Realistic, Time-bound
SWOT	Strengths, Weaknesses, Opportunities, Threats
WBL	work based learning

PART

1 Introducing work based learning

How does learning happen in the workplace?

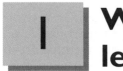

What is work based learning?

Tom Aird

Introduction

You may have chosen to undertake a course to help you learn at work for your career progression, and this may be a Foundation Degree (FD). FDs help you to learn at work, for work, in order to enhance your skill base, your role, the quality of care you provide, your future employability and your ability to learn throughout your career, which is otherwise known as lifelong learning (LLL). This learning at work, for work, is referred to as work based learning (WBL). Therefore, to make the most of your studies, it is important that you understand the concept of WBL. You may initially find WBL difficult and challenging. This may be related to your preferred learning styles, and previous experiences of being on a course; however, one of the skills you will develop is learning how to learn on the job. Learning happens at work every day; however, in a busy, demanding work environment we do not always acknowledge the learning which takes place.

This chapter aims to help you understand the concept of WBL and how to make the most of learning while doing your FD. Upon completion of this chapter, you should be able to do the following:

1 Define the concepts of WBL and LLL;

2 Understand the importance of LLL for you;

3 Identify the role of WBL in your workplace.

What is work based learning?

In this section we explore definitions of WBL and provide you with some activities that will help you understand how this relates to your course or workplace. In addition, it explores the link between WBL and lifelong learning.

The phrase 'work based learning' is often used to describe a unit of study that has a significant workplace element to it. For example, in your FD, you may have workplace tasks to complete that help you to learn on the job. There may be a course component that requires you and your manager to identify your learning needs and plan activities to meet those needs either in the classroom or in the workplace.

WBL differs from traditional classroom learning because it is centred on reflection on your work and occurs following some sort of action or problem-solving within your working environment. This is known as **action learning**. Action learning is a method for individual and organizational development. Working in small groups, people tackle important organizational issues or problems and learn from their attempts to change things. Action learning brings people together to exchange, support and challenge each other in seeking to act and learn. Action learning on an FD course enables you to meet in small groups with other students or workplace colleagues to discuss and explore workplace problems and attempt to reach practical solutions. This type of learning requires new knowledge and developing the skill of learning how to learn in the workplace (Raelin 2000).

Fatima, an FD graduate, comments on her experiences of using action learning.

As a small group from different workplaces we chose to meet on a regular basis at the university to discuss areas which we had covered in class. I found this really beneficial as it allowed me to ask questions and share experiences in a safe environment.

The benefits of action learning for an FD student include:

- increasing your self-awareness and ability to identify personal development challenges;
- enabling you to engage in a voyage of discovery and enquiry with your peers in order to solve problems or issues;
- helping you to relate to other people and communicate more effectively;
- encouraging you to think reflectively, creatively and critically in achieving solutions to problems or issues;
- helping you to develop initiative and readiness to take responsibility for your actions;
- helping you to challenge the status quo and the 'normal way of doing things around here' in order to effect change;
- providing peer support, encouragement and collaboration;
- enabling individuals and teams to learn while working;
- encouraging the development of leadership skills in participants who take on different roles and responsibilities within the group to reach solutions to different problems or issues.

Chapter 2 explores the concept of action learning in more detail and the role that reflection plays in promoting learning at work is discussed in Chapter 4.

Your FD course is specifically designed to meet your needs as a learner and contribute to the longer-term development of your workplace. Each individual student on your course will have very specific individual learning needs. Your individual needs should reflect what knowledge and skills you must learn in order to undertake your work role as well as any specific areas of personal development which you identify. To help you explore the differences in learning needs among your fellow learners, undertake the following Time Out activities:

Time Out: Understanding differing learning needs across organizations

Find someone within your group who is employed in a different role from you. Discuss what their individual learning needs are and compare these to your own. How similar or how different are they?

You are likely to be employed in an organization which is continuously undergoing change. As a consequence, the organization must respond to these changes and this can only happen through a skilled and knowledgeable, flexible workforce.

In your workplace, can you identify its vision, goals and priorities for the future? Now compare these with other students on your course – does the workplace vision identify the importance of learning and the need for a skilled workforce?

How does work based learning feature in your Foundation Degree?

Your FD will consist of a portfolio of activities designed to meet four key types of learning (Brennan 2007: 20):

- *Learning at work* – learning that takes place in the workplace.

- *Learning through work* – learning while working.

- *Learning for work* – learning how to do new or existing things better.

- *Learning from work* – learning from the experience of work.

For example, you may already have experience of working in your current role and have learned from that experience *at work*. In conjunction with this, you constantly refine the skills you have developed and are learning *through work*. The FD course may include a module which is taught in the classroom and where you will learn *for work*. Supporting this may be a WBL module which will help you draw the theoretical and practical elements together allowing you to learn *from work*.

How does your FD enable you to meet learning outcomes?

Your FD course will use a variety of methods to help you achieve both the prescribed course and your own individually negotiated learning outcomes. A **learning outcome** is a statement of what you are expected to know, understand and/or be able to do at the end of a period of learning. Learning outcomes are generally written to reflect four areas of learning:

- *knowledge* (demonstrate knowledge and understanding of ...);

- *cognitive skills* (describe, compare, evaluate, apply, etc.);

- *subject-specific skills* (co-ordinates, balances, operates, handles, performs, calibrates, etc.);

- *key skills* (these may be academic and/or technical skills defined by the university and the workplace).

At the beginning of your FD, the aim is to help you identify the knowledge and skills which you already have. This allows you to identify your prior learning and look back on the career journey you have taken so far. It acts as a vital starting point in the preparation for future learning at work. One of the most obvious ways that this is often demonstrated is through the use of a portfolio of learning. A portfolio is a useful tool to enable you to demonstrate significant areas of learning and professional competence derived from all formal and informal learning opportunities in the workplace. The portfolio is a compilation of learning intentions, accounts of learning activities, learning outcomes and records of reflective dialogues. Your portfolio can include evidence such as certificates, statements from colleagues, course work already completed and your Personal Development Plan or appraisal from your workplace. This is discussed in more depth in Chapters 6 and 7. The Time Out activity below will help you explore this further.

Time Out: Identifying your learning

Review your curriculum vitae and write down your key achievements and areas of learning in different jobs or activities you have been involved with.

Simon, a first year FD student, shares his experiences of identifying his key achievements and the impact this has had on his own learning:

On the first day of my Foundation Degree I was asked to consider areas where I felt learning had occurred while undertaking my workplace role. At the time I could not see the relevance of this activity but, as I have progressed through the first year of the Foundation Degree I can see how important it was in enabling me to understand how I learn.

Once you have identified what you need to learn, your FD course will require you to negotiate with your course tutor and/or employer what additional knowledge and skills you need to learn. It is very important that you have a clear focus of your learning priorities through the development of a **learning contract**. Learning contracts provide a formal framework for structuring your learning activities. For further detail about learning contracts, see Chapter 4. Your learning is personal to you and WBL enables you to customize what you need to know, through the identification of your personal needs, in order to fulfil your workplace role both now and in the future. The Time Out activity below will help you identify your learning needs.

Time Out: Identifying areas for development

Review your current job description and write down which areas you need to develop to carry out your role more effectively and efficiently.

It is really important that once you have identified your learning, you are able to explain how this learning has occurred. This will be achieved through report writing, essays and project work as examples. There may be further opportunity for you to identify when learning has not gone to plan. In this instance, you may be given opportunities to make recommendations for future learning which you can revisit and evaluate in your PDP. Chapter 7 explores personal development planning in more detail.

How does work based learning contribute to your lifelong learning (LLL)?

The concept of lifelong learning is based upon the principle that formal learning takes place throughout your life, it does not stop because you have completed a course. Table 1.1 lists some of the differences between traditional approaches to learning and LLL.

Table 1.1 Differences between traditional approaches to learning and those of lifelong learning

Traditional approaches to learning	Approaches to lifelong learning
Content driven by the tutor, relates to information giving in the classroom, i.e. lectures	Based on the learners' needs in relation to their occupational role. The learning experience is negotiated between the learner, their employer and tutor, and agreed in the form of learning objectives
The teacher is in control of what learning should take place	The student is in control of what learning should take place
Didactic, rote learning, learning may be superficial	Uses methods such as action learning, problem solving, reflection, so deeper meaningful learning takes place
The learner is a passive recipient in the learning process	The learner is an active recipient in the learning process

LLL helps you to enhance your career and update your skills and capabilities to remain employable. LLL enables you to create programmes of study around priorities set by your work, career aspirations or personal interests. This ultimately promotes and helps you to develop skills in independent learning and moves away from the notion that lifelong learning is course dependent. To achieve this, you need to be motivated and develop skills and strategies to become a self-directed learner. Developing your own motivation to learn throughout your career is very important for LLL and we explore this further in Chapters 3 and 9.

What factors can affect the quality of your learning in the workplace?

Having discussed how your FD course is designed to promote WBL, we now turn our attention to the factors which affect the quality of your learning in the workplace.

Learning in the workplace is dependent upon the range of experiences available, the quality of support you are offered by colleagues, access to workplace supervision, your previous experience and your preferred learning styles. Workplace learning experiences need to be sufficient enough to meet the outcomes of the course which you are studying and your own development needs. In Chapters 2 and 3 we explore the impact that workplace culture has in the learning environment and in turn the impact this has on you.

Who will support you during your course?

The most important aspect of learning in the workplace is the human dimension whereby learning is facilitated in an atmosphere of mutual respect and cooperation between you, your employer (work based mentor) and your tutor. Your employer is central to the success of any WBL initiatives. They have first-hand knowledge and understanding of the complexities of your workplace and are best placed to guide you when choosing a suitable work based mentor. Try the Time Out activities below to help you explore your relationship with your employer and their support of your WBL initiatives.

Time Out: Supporting learning in the workplace

Reflect on your role in the workplace and think about the following points:

- **What have you learnt in the past six months?**
- **How did your employer help you to achieve this learning?**

In discussion with fellow students, identify how variable workplace experiences can impact on your learning:

- **What are the positives of your collective experiences?**
- **What are the challenging aspects of your collective experiences?**
- **From this discussion, what do you consider supports effective learning in the workplace?**

Following completion of these activities, Table 1.2 provides a summary of features which promote effective WBL. Chapter 2 further explores the role of the student and employer in creating a supportive learning environment in the workplace.

As you can see from the Time Out activities, effective team work is essential to the success of your WBL in the classroom and in the workplace. To this end, it is important that individual roles and responsibilities are clearly understood. As a WBL student you need to:

- identify your learning needs through reflection and joint appraisal/negotiation with your work-based mentor and tutor;

- record your personal and professional progress regularly;

- use opportunities to learn in the workplace and reflect upon these in a timely manner, integrating new knowledge into practice;

- provide evidence of achievement of personal, professional and workplace practice where required;

- maintain confidentiality at all times.

Table 1.2 Organizational readiness checklist for work based learning activities

Organizational Readiness Checklist	Yes	No
1. Learning is incorporated into everything people do.		
2. Learning for learning's sake is encouraged and rewarded.		
3. The organization supports teamwork, creativity, empowerment and quality.		
4. Employees are trusted and encouraged to choose courses that they need.		
5. People with different job titles from different departments learn together.		
6. The organization promotes mentoring relationships to enhance learning.		
7. Learning is an integral part of meetings, work groups, and work processes.		
8. Everyone in the organization has equal access to learning.		
9. Mistakes are learning opportunities.		
10. The organization encourages cross-training and rewards employees.		

Source: Johnson (2001).

As part of your FD course you should have identified a work based mentor whose role is to provide regular support and guidance within the workplace. They should help you to integrate theory you have learnt in the classroom with your roles and responsibilities in the workplace. They should provide an opportunity to directly observe your work so that they can report your progress regularly to you and your tutor. They therefore have a key role in assessing, monitoring and evaluating your learning. The role of the mentor is discussed in more detail in Chapter 7.

Similarly, your course tutor has responsibilities for supporting guided reflection and action learning, helping you to integrate classroom learning with workplace activities. Their role is to assess the evidence you provide, liaise with your mentor on a regular basis to evaluate your progress and to make sure your workplace can support the range of WBL activities your course requires.

One of the challenges in this relationship for you might be your dual role as employee and WBL student. Durrant, Rhodes and Young (2009: 34) highlight some of the ethical issues associated with WBL. They state: 'Unlike campus based students, the ethical issues are likely to be more complex and more significant because the work-based learner operates within workplace, occupational and sometimes professional contexts.' Access in the workplace to confidential and sensitive information, insider knowledge of the organization, honesty and deception, confidentiality, intellectual property and plagiarism are some of the issues they acknowledge. It is really important, therefore, that you set some ground rules with your employer and course tutor at the beginning of your course, perhaps at the time you are writing your learning contract.

In summary, this chapter has introduced you to the concept of WBL and how you can identify and make the most of learning in the workplace to meet your individual development needs. In Chapter 2 we will discuss how workplace culture affects your learning at work.

Key learning points

- WBL focuses on helping you to learn at work, from work, for work to enable you to perform your role to the best of your ability and provide high quality care.

- WBL focuses on learning through reflection following some sort of action or problem solving within the working environment to reach practical solutions.

- Your individual learning needs are personal to you and are shaped by your past experience, career history, workplace role and type of service you provide.

- Your FD course provides structured learning activities to achieve both prescribed and personally set learning outcomes.

- Learning contracts and portfolios of learning should be negotiated with your course tutor and workplace mentor who will work in partnership with you to achieve your objectives.

- Optimal learning takes place when you build good relationships with workplace colleagues, your mentor and your course tutor, and enables you to understand roles and responsibilities in the learning process.

- Developing skills and strategies to increase your ability to direct your own learning will enhance your career and your motivation as a lifelong learner.

Critical review questions

1 How can work based learning help you in the development of your occupational role?
2 How are your personal development needs met in your current job?
3 How do you envisage your career developing over the next five years?

Web links and resources

Department of Health.
http://www.dh.gov.uk/en/index.htm

Lifelong Learning.
http://www.lifelonglearning.co.uk/

Skills for Health.
http://www.skillsforhealth.org.uk/

Reading for interest

Raelin, J. (2008) *Work-Based Learning: Bridging Knowledge and Action in the Workplace*. Chichester: John Wiley & Sons, Ltd.

Rounce, K. and Workman, B. (eds) (2005) *Work-based Learning in Health Care: Applications and Innovations*. Chichester: Kingsham.

References

Brennan, L. (2007) What is the higher education work-based learning 'product'?, in L. Brennan and D. Hemsworth (eds) *Incorporating into Higher Education Programmes the Learning People do for, in and through Work*. Bolton: University Vocational Awards Council.

Durrant, A., Rhodes, G. and Young, D. (eds) (2009) *Getting Started with University-Level Work Based Learning*. London: Middlesex University Press.

Johnson, D. (2001) The opportunities, benefits and barriers to the introduction of work-based learning in higher education. *Innovations in Education and Teaching International*, 38(4), 364–68.

Raelin, J.A. (2000) *Work-based Learning: The New Frontier of Management Development*. Englewood Cliffs, NJ: Prentice Hall.

2 | How does learning happen in the workplace?

Carolyn Jackson

Introduction

Chapter 1 identified how WBL occurs through the activity of solving real problems either on your own, through structured activities or through working with a group of colleagues either in a classroom environment or in the workplace. This chapter explores the concept of learning further, focusing on the ways in which you learn at work, the impact that workplace culture has on your ability to learn, and the role those members of the multi-disciplinary team play in supporting your development. It will help you to understand the importance of being aware of your learning needs, and emphasize the importance of being structured in how you plan to make the most of opportunities that arise to develop your career. It provides a range of activities to help you focus on questioning yourself and your approach to learning.

Upon completion of this chapter, you should be able to do the following:

1 identify how learning occurs in the workplace;

2 explain the role of action learning and experiential learning in the workplace;

3 describe the impact of workplace culture and colleagues and peers on your own learning;

4 outline a clear plan of how to make the most of your own learning opportunities at work.

How do we define learning?

The importance of learning was first put forward by a Chinese philosopher, Confucius (551–479 BC). He believed that everyone should benefit from learning: 'Without learning, the wise become foolish; by learning, the foolish become wise.'

We use the term learning to describe the way an individual, and indeed a workplace, builds, reorganizes and changes the way knowledge is used and applied to different situations or activities. The term knowledge refers to facts, theories, procedures, social skills, strategies, worldviews (the way you look at the world and understand it), and values of the workplace – the kind of 'stuff' you know at work. Some people think of knowledge as a possession, others define it as an activity. The fact that you might work in a knowledge-rich environment does not mean that you will automatically acquire new knowledge. Knowledge is engaged only when you attend to it, use it to perform an action, display it or otherwise operate on it. What really matters is the nature of your participation in workplace activities that might promote learning and strengthen your knowledge base.

According to Gerber (1998), there are 11 ways by which you can learn at work:

1 by making mistakes and learning not to repeat them;

2 through self-education on and off the job;

3 through practising personal values;

4 by applying theory and practising skills;

5 through solving problems;

6 through interacting with others;

7 through open lateral planning;

8 by being an advocate for colleagues, for example, through staff committees;

9 through offering leadership to others;

10 through formal training;

11 through practising quality assurance.

There are hundreds of learning theories but the one most relevant to the workplace is that of action learning.

What is action learning?

Action learning is an umbrella term used to describe a set of activities that, according to Cusins (1995), 'create a context for creative decision making in uncertain situations'.

These activities include:

1 *Experiential learning* – **experiential learning** theory seeks to help you integrate theory from your course into your workplace practice to create, test and refine the knowledge and skills you need to do your job. This is often referred to as *professional/craft knowledge*. An important part of experiential learning is the ability to reflect in and on practice (this will be discussed in more depth in Chapters 3–5). Your course will enable you to develop skills required for disciplined reflection to enable you to make sense of knowledge gained and apply this learning to a range of different situations.

2 *Creative problem solving* – is an important aspect of action learning because it enables you to define and make sense of practical issues, generate a range of different solutions and apply the most appropriate one to your practice.

3 *Acquiring relevant knowledge* – from a range of different sources such as colleagues, books, journals, policies, procedures or the internet.

4 *Peer group support* – you learn from each other's experiences as a resource which in turn enables you to make more informed decisions in your practice.

One of the most important aspects of action learning is your ability to take responsibility for your own learning, to learn from problems at hand which are relevant to your everyday practice. You need to be able to question your everyday practice to develop a better understanding of the functions, skills, knowledge, and processes needed to solve daily activities. This requires you to find out what you need to know/learn as well as understanding what you already know and how to apply this knowledge to the workplace. In essence, only you can identify what you need to learn, others are there to support you as a resource. Action learning builds on the relationship between reflection and action. It is an approach to WBL which enables you to meet others from your course in small groups to discuss and explore problems and attempt to reach an appropriate solution. If you are not undertaking a course, you may meet regularly with colleagues or peers through perhaps a team meeting or for some readers, through a journal club, a research interest group or some other clinical standards working group. The important thing here is that meeting regularly as a group helps you to evaluate and learn from real workplace problems.

When we learn, we rely on the context in which instruction occurs to determine the usefulness and meaning of knowledge and this is critical to your ability to transfer that knowledge to new situations (Brown et al. 1989). As an FD student you may find yourself as a novice learner if you have not undertaken any further study for some time.

Simon, a first year FD student shares his experiences of being a novice.

I can still remember my first day at university, my knees trembled, my mouth was dry and my stomach was churning. What was I doing at university? University is for people with A levels, not those who had left school with minimal formal qualifications. Our tutor tried to reassure us that we had expertise in the workplace and that we would be supported to develop the required academic skills. At first I was not sure, but as soon as I began to realize the academic requirements, my confidence grew as I had the workplace experience.

Simon raises the important issue of seeking out support from course tutors, workplace mentors and fellow students. This is explored in more detail in Chapters 1 and 4 through to 7. At this point, however, it is important to mention the worth of finding a suitable workplace mentor to help you acquire and apply the knowledge you learn on your course. Your workplace mentor should be able to help you learn conceptual, factual, procedural and self-management strategies as well as the tricks of the trade.

How does the culture of your workplace influence your learning?

The culture of your workplace is extremely influential on your ability to learn and to be supported to develop your role, responsibilities and career aspirations. Your workplace culture affects whether and how readily you can gain access to particular kinds of knowledge. The environment in which you learn is governed by what is commonly known as the *micro politics of knowledge* – who gets to know what, who controls that knowledge, and how it is used. It is available to you personally or as a group only when it is used or displayed in a context in which you actively participate. There are many methods for capturing knowledge and experience, such as publications, activity reports, lessons learned, interviews, and presentations. Capturing includes organizing knowledge in ways that people can find it; multiple structures facilitate searches regardless of the user's perspective (e.g. who, what, when, where, why, and how). Capturing also includes storage in repositories, databases, or libraries to ensure that the knowledge will be available when and as needed.

Try the following Time Out activity to consider the knowledge and experience held by your colleagues in the workplace and the impact this has on your own learning.

Time Out: What impact do the knowledge and experience of your colleagues have on your own learning?

- **Review your current role: identify the number of staff in different occupational roles who work alongside you.**
- **What knowledge and experience do they make available to you in the workplace?**
- **Do they freely share this knowledge?**
- **If not, who holds the knowledge you require and how can you access it?**
- **Is it the person who you expect it to be, if not, why not?**

If your workplace readily shares knowledge and is committed to learning both for itself and for its workforce, it is referred to as a **learning organization**. A learning organization accepts and adapts readily to new ideas and changes and has a shared vision and collective goals for development (Pedlar et al. 1997). It demonstrates a continuous ability to learn and adapt to the changing needs of society. This is important because health and social care services need to respond to and adapt to the changing health needs of local communities and government priorities.

Harrison (2000) suggests that the everyday experience of work and the need to continually cope with change in the workplace have the most influential bearing on what people learn. It is therefore the culture of the workplace which promotes effective WBL. The culture of your workplace influences the way in which your colleagues behave and is linked to the values, beliefs and human action and activities within your organization (Schein 1985).

An effective workplace culture that promotes your learning has four key characteristics:

1 It demonstrates a holistic person-centred approach to patients, service users and staff.

2 It promotes daily decision-making that is transparent and draws on evidence from all the knowledge necessary for effective person-centred care, e.g. evidence from rigorous research, critical reflection and professional expertise and local knowledge.

3 It focuses on personal, individual, team and service effectiveness. It promotes a culture of lifelong learning and ensures that it critiques and evaluates the quality of its service and the support it offers its workforce on a regular basis;

4 It is committed to the development of future leaders within the workplace by encouraging its staff to own and learn from improvements and innovations in practice.

If we break these characteristics down further, an effective learning environment within your workplace should demonstrate:

- a collective vision, values and mission statement realized in practice;

- a commitment to person-centred practice and a concern for the quality of care provided;

- a commitment to team work, collaborative decision-making, inclusion and participation;

- an understanding of the roles and responsibilities of individual team members and of the collective responsibility of the multi-disciplinary team;

- adaptability, innovation and creativity to maintain workplace effectiveness and evidence that change is driven by the needs of patients/users/communities;

- recognized formal systems to evaluate learning and development, performance and quality of service delivery (Manley 2004).

In order for this to happen, the workplace should demonstrate a range of supportive learning strategies and take a broad view of learning and development activities to enable you to meet the needs of your role. You can identify this in your workplace through evidence such as tailored personal development plans, a mentor network to provide support for learning in the workplace and recognition of learning achieved. The following Time Out activity will enable you to explore the common features of your own workplace culture.

Time Out: Common features of your workplace culture

- **How would you describe your workplace culture?**
- **What are the core values that are most talked about at work?**
- **What are the values that are actually experienced by your patients, their families, yourself and your colleagues?**
- **What examples can you give of opportunities to learn from colleagues in your multi-disciplinary team?**

How do your colleagues influence your learning at work?

Creating (or acquiring) knowledge can be an individual or group activity. However, as first stated by Lucilius in the first century BC: 'Knowledge is not knowledge until someone else knows that one knows.'

At work, your colleagues are an important source of learning and support. You work with a range of health and social care practitioners (a multi-disciplinary team) in a workplace community and should have a shared vision, values and goals for the quality of service you provide for your patients and their families. There should be a commitment to partnership ways of working and learning from each other. It is important that you understand what impact the multi-disciplinary team has on sharing and producing knowledge and learning opportunities, and tap into these to promote opportunities to maximize your own learning.

An effective multi-disciplinary team should value the contributions that all individuals and team members make in planning every aspect of care around the patient and their family, and views care in relation to how health care and social care needs fit into the context of the person's life plan. It should be able to adapt internally and externally to change, reflected by a learning culture so that team members learn from each other and should value the opinions of its members. It should be committed to matching the service to the needs of its local community population.

Fatima, a graduate FD student, remarks on how important the multi-disciplinary team was to her learning:

I was very lucky when I started my programme because I was working in a very progressive service where the multi-disciplinary team had good strong relationships and valued the importance of learning together to improve the quality of care.

At the start of my course, my workplace mentor encouraged me to discuss my learning needs with a variety of different team members. I shadowed members of the team in order to gain greater insight into and understanding of the roles they undertake, and the responsibilities they have to their client groups. This in turn helped me to understand how a combination of different professional roles, skills and expertise can contribute to effective team working.

I would recommend to any FD student to work with different members of their team while studying in the workplace to enhance their understanding of what can be learned from other professional groups.

How can you make the most of learning opportunities in the workplace?

In order to make the most of learning opportunities in the workplace, it is important that you have an understanding of your own learning styles and preferences and an appreciation of the sorts of toolkits that are available to support your learning and development. You might like to have a look at Chapters 3–6 for practical support and guidance.

So what can you do to promote your own learning in the workplace? Here we identify a range of strategies you might use to make the most of learning opportunities both during your course and in the workplace.

1 *Be organized if you are undertaking a course of study*. You should be clear about the aims and objectives of your course and each module that you are undertaking. This information is available in your course handbook, through course online materials, and from your personal or module tutors. Be sure that you ask questions during your induction to the course if you are not clear about how the course relates to your workplace and your role. Be clear about the tutor's, your employer's and your own expectations, roles and responsibilities so that you can maximize learning opportunities. Identifying problems early on will enable you to find workable solutions before it becomes a major issue and seemingly unmanageable.

2 *Have a clear study plan that maps out what you need to learn and how you relate assignments to the workplace*. This should include time for reading, writing and balancing this against work and family commitments. A learning contract designed with your tutor's support will enable you to achieve this. Similarly, having developed a study plan for your home life will enable you to have designated study time if you are balancing family, work and life commitments with your course.

3 *Hold regular meetings with your course tutors to check your progress and to discuss areas that you may be experiencing difficulty with*. This enables you to acknowledge and celebrate success as well as identifying areas where you may need further support or development time.

4 *Read regularly in the library or online to ensure you are keeping your learning current and are aware of the latest evidence and thinking in the field*. This will help you to build your self-confidence and self-esteem when applying this learning to the workplace as you will be able to justify the evidence base underpinning the care you deliver.

5 *Schedule regular meetings with your manager/workplace mentor to review your learning objectives and personal development plan*. This should achieve similar outcomes to the meetings with your tutors.

6 *Try to identify opportunities to work closely with the multi-disciplinary team to understand different types of professional knowledge used in everyday practice*. The opportunity to debrief with colleagues will help you unpack what knowledge has informed the decisions taken by the team in care delivery.

7 *Take opportunities to gain feedback from your patients/clients/service users and colleagues*. This may be difficult to achieve but is worth pursuing. You can find different types or sources of evidence to help you achieve this. Some examples include: (i) talking to your patients and their families to gain their views of the quality of care they have received; (ii) using patient survey tools to understand how patient groups perceive the quality of a range of different care services; (iii) talking to patient liaison services or patient action groups; (iv) getting feedback from your colleagues either verbally in coffee discussions or by using peer review survey tools available as part of your appraisal process; and (v) gaining informal feedback and support from your peer group on your course.

Thinking further about these tips and strategies look at the following Time Out activity and think about how this might help you form a plan for your course.

Time Out: Creating a study plan

- **Draw up an initial plan of study to create a balance between study, work and family life.**
- **Who would you identify as your workplace mentor and why?**
- **What qualities do they possess to support your learning?**
- **What opportunities are there for you to push the boundaries of your learning?**
- **Can you think about situations you would like to be involved in that are challenging?**
- **How will you deal with constructive feedback that might not always be positive?**

This chapter has introduced you to the characteristics of an effective learning environment and the role of colleagues in supporting your learning in the workplace. In Chapter 3, we will discuss how your learning style affects the way you learn.

Key learning points

- We have described learning as the way a workplace builds, reorganizes and changes the way knowledge is used and applied to different situations or activities. The term knowledge refers to facts, theories, procedures, social skills, strategies, worldviews (the way you look at the world and understand it), and values of the workplace – the kind of 'stuff' you know at work.

- Knowledge gained through and in workplace practice stems from a variety of structured activities, creative thinking in uncertain situations to solve everyday problems, reflection on action with colleagues and peers, and through structured education courses or programmes.

- The culture of a workplace impacts both positively and negatively on the value placed on learning and development. Learning organizations promote knowledge exchange, and place learning and development at the core of their values in order to adapt to a constantly changing health and social care context.

- An effective learning environment will include a commitment to person-centred practice, a shared vision, a concern for the quality of care provided, a commitment to team work, a lifelong learning culture and the systems of formal critique and evaluation to underpin this.

- The multi-disciplinary team is an important source of learning and support and an effective understanding of how it works in your workplace community will help you make the most of opportunities to enhance your professional development.

- You can make the most of learning opportunities in the workplace by being organized, developing a clear study plan and drawing upon regular support and feedback from managers, peers, mentors and course tutors as well as service users.

Critical review questions

- What knowledge and skills do you believe you need to develop in order to be more effective in the workplace?
- Are there any potential barriers to your learning and development and, if so, how might these be overcome?
- What does your study plan indicate as possible sources of learning and development either through formal (courses) or informal (workplace learning) mechanisms?
- Who do you work well with in the workplace and how might you approach them to support you as a workplace mentor should you be considering further study through perhaps a Foundation Degree?

Web links and resources

Information about university courses that help you learn direct.
www.learningthroughwork.org

Information and advice about NHS careers.
www.nhscareers.nhs.uk

Information about national benchmark standards for Assistant/Associate Practitioners.
www.skillsforhealth.org.uk

Reading for interest

Durrant, A., Rhodes, G. and Young, D. (eds) (2009) *Getting Started with University-Level Work Based Learning*. London: Middlesex University Press.
Jasper, M. (2006) *Professional Development, Reflection, and Decision Making*. Oxford: Blackwell.
McGill, I. and Brockbank, A. (2004) *The Action Learning Handbook*. London: Routledge Falmer.

References

Brown, J.S., Collins, A. and Duguid, P. (1989) Situated cognition and the culture of learning. *Educational Researcher*, 18(1): 32–42.
Cusins, P. (1995) Action learning revisited. *Industrial and Commercial Training*, 27(4): 3–10.
Gerber, R. (1998) How do workers learn in their work? *The Learning Organization*, 5(4): 168–75.
Harrison, R. (2000) Employee development. 2nd edition. London: Chartered Institute of Personnel Development.

Manley, K. (2004) Workplace culture: is your workplace effective? How would you know? Editorial. British Association of Critical Care Nurses, *Nursing in Critical Care*, 9(1): 1–3.

Pedlar, M., Burgogyne, J. and Boydell, T. (1997) *The Learning Company: A Strategy for Sustainable Development*, 2nd edn. London: McGraw-Hill.

Schein, E.H. (1985) *Organizational Culture and Leadership*. San Francisco, CA: Jossey-Bass.

3 How does your learning style affect your ability to learn in the workplace?

Barbara Workman

Introduction

Many people who undertake a work based learning (WBL) programme find it a big adjustment in their work to become both a worker and a learner. It requires new skills; not just new knowledge, but also the development of a deeper understanding of yourself; how you learn, what motivates you to learn and how to make connections between theories and practical skills. It involves exploiting and recognizing available learning opportunities.

Upon completion of this chapter, you should be able to do the following:

1 Demonstrate an understanding of your personal learning styles and preferences.

2 Identify how your personality influences your preferred learning style.

3 Understand the difference between deep and surface learning.

4 Understand different methods of learning in the workplace.

Why is an understanding of your personal learning style and preferences important?

You may have chosen to undertake a WBL course because you do not want to follow a traditional academic route of study. This may be for a number of reasons, but it might be that the thought of being in a classroom all day either frustrates or frightens you. Previous experiences at school often influence how you learn as an adult, and many adults prefer not to study after they have left school because past failures have undermined their confidence, or they do not feel clever, or have failed important exams. It is worth realizing that not everyone who passes exams is especially intelligent, but they may have a good memory, or just learn exam techniques. Intelligence takes a number of different forms and most of us are good at some things and not others. Discovering how you learn is a way to find new confidence and skills. So, to start with, you may have to face some of your study demons! You should consider these now because you have chosen a course that expects you to study at university level as well as work. However, it may feel easier for you to avoid studying by cleaning the house from top to bottom or doing overtime! Even people who do academic work find ways to avoid it when they are unsure what is needed, or are not really motivated. The key word here is 'motivation' for learning. Try the following Time Out activity to understand what motivates you.

Time Out: What motivates you to learn?

- **What is it that will motivate you through your course?**
- **What is it that excites you about this course?**
- **How will it help you in three or five years time?**

Make a list of the pros and cons of doing your course as a worker and a learner:

- **Are these likely to change?**
- **If so, are there any you can change now to make sure you can stick with it?**

Record these thoughts to remind yourself that there are some very important reasons why you have chosen this course. Your personal motivation as an adult will see you through the course. Once you have identified your motivation for WBL, it will help you to get the best out of it.

Your learning style is as individual as your personality and is your personal preference for learning. Knowing your personality and how you respond to other people is an important aspect of becoming a professional, and understanding yourself and others. You can discover whether you are an extrovert or introvert and if you make decisions based on your feelings, intuition, senses, perceptions or facts. For example, extroverts recharge their batteries by socializing and mixing with lots of people, and introverts like to refresh themselves by being quiet and alone. You may wonder how this affects learning. By knowing your personality preferences, you can find ways to learn from colleagues or clients to experience better learning opportunities. For example, if you are an introvert, but your mentor is an extrovert, and likes to teach in a noisy, busy environment, you may find that it is too distracting to concentrate. By understanding that it is a personality preference, it makes it easier to ask if you could go to a quieter place with fewer distractions. To help you find out more about your personality type go to the following websites which provide you with assessment tools that identify your personality:

- http://www.humanmetrics.com/cgi-win/JTypes2.asp

- http://www.myersbriggs.org/type-use-for-everyday-life/

It can be fun to do and may help you understand your family members or friends better too!

Fatima, a graduate FD student, shares how she benefitted from knowing her personality type.

Our tutor suggested that there are different ways to determine what our preferred learning styles are through assessment tools that help to highlight your personality type. I did not really know why this was but I was curious to discover more. I am really pleased that I invested the time and energy to undertake this activity because I learnt that I was an introvert. Understanding my personality type helped me to understand that I have a different way of approaching my learning as I am a quiet learner. I had experienced some initial problems with my mentor who is a very outgoing person and has an extrovert personality. This assessment helped me to realize why I could not always work well with my mentor and it gave me the confidence to discuss this with my mentor to find a way to work effectively together to enhance my learning and meet my learning needs.

As well as different tools to understand your personality type, there are also a range of tools to allow you to identify your preferred learning styles, and two models will be discussed in this section: Honey and Mumford's learning styles and Visual, Auditory, Reading and Kinaesthetic (VARK) learning styles. Understanding your learning style will strengthen your weaker learning preferences so that you can take advantage of more learning opportunities and solve problems more effectively. It will also help you to understand how others learn and why things that work for you do not necessarily work for others.

Honey and Mumford's learning styles

Honey and Mumford (2006) identified four different types of learners: activists, reflectors, pragmatists and theorists. Most people are a mixture of these but with particular preferences. Honey and Mumford's learning styles are discussed below. If you want to know more about these or find out your own learning style, you can visit www.peterhoney.com or ask your tutor, as many courses have access to it. To encourage you to explore these four types of learning, you might like to try this Time Out activity while you are reading through the descriptions:

Time Out: Types of learning

Consider Honey and Mumford's four different learning styles.

- **Which ones can you identify with?**
- **Can you relate any to colleagues or clients?**
- **How might that make a difference to you when you work with them?**

Make some notes of any insights this exercise has given you. These can contribute to your learning during your course and/or within the workplace.

The Activist

Honey and Mumford (2006) state:

Activists like to take direct action. They are enthusiastic and welcome new challenges and experiences. They are less interested in what has happened in the past or in putting new things into a broader context. They are primarily interested in the here and now. They like to have a go, try things out and participate. They like to be the centre of attention.

To summarize, Activists like:

- to think on their feet;
- to have short sessions;
- plenty of variety;
- the opportunity to initiate;
- to participate and have fun.

This means that Activists learn less when:

- analysing and interpreting data;
- passively listening to lectures or reading long articles;
- working or studying alone.

Learning approaches that Activists can develop include:

- pondering past events and planning future activities;
- observing and listening to others as they lead activities;
- staying with one activity longer before rushing to the next.

The Reflector

Honey and Mumford (2006) describe Reflectors as people who:

like to think about things in detail before taking action. They take a thoughtful approach. They are good listeners and prefer to adopt a low profile. They are prepared to read and re-read and will welcome the opportunity to repeat a piece of learning.

To summarize, Reflectors like:

- to think before acting;
- thorough preparation;
- to research and evaluate;
- to make decisions in their own time;
- to listen and observe.

Consequently they learn less from:

- taking action without planning;
- being rushed into new things or working to tight deadlines;
- being a leader.

Learning approaches that Reflectors can develop include:

- using structured study skills to maximize their time;
- actively participating in an event rather than observing;
- making a decision based on partial information.

The Theorist

Honey and Mumford (2006) describe Theorists as individuals who:

> like to see how things fit into an overall pattern. They are logical and objective systems people who prefer a sequential approach to problems. They are analytical, pay great attention to detail and tend to be perfectionists.

To summarize, Theorists like:

- concepts and models;
- to see the overall picture;
- to feel intellectually stretched;
- structure and clear objectives;
- logical presentation of ideas.

If you are a Theorist, you will learn less from:

- unstructured activities which are uncertain or ambiguous;
- situations involving emotions and feelings;
- taking action without a clear rationale or principle.

Learning approaches that Theorists can develop include:

- thinking 'out of the box';
- reflection on events and keeping a learning diary;
- considering ideas and thoughts of others.

The Pragmatist

Honey and Mumford's (2006) describe Pragmatists as individuals who:

> like to see how things work in practice. They enjoy experimenting with new ideas. They are practical, down to earth and like to solve problems. They appreciate the opportunity to try out what they have learned/are learning.

To summarize, Pragmatists like:

- to see the relevance of their work;
- to gain practical advantage from learning;
- credible role models;
- proven techniques;
- activities to be real.

This means that Pragmatists learn less from:

- lack of evidence of immediate benefit to the situation or apparent irrelevance;
- people who appear distant from the real issues;
- theoretical events with no practical application.

Learning approaches that Pragmatists can develop include:

- identifying and completing priorities and goals;
- analysis and critical thinking to construct an argument;
- lateral thinking and understanding alternative views.

Visual, Auditory, Reading, Kinaesthetic Learning Styles (VARK)

Another popular approach to learning styles is called **VARK**: Visual, Auditory, Reading/Writing and Kinaesthetic (touch). VARK is a questionnaire that provides a quick and easy evaluation of your preferred learning style and preferences. The aim is to get you thinking about the process of learning. Being a good 'student' is about learning to learn, it is a set of skills that are learnt and improve with practice. Like anything else, it takes time, commitment and a little help from your friends.

Visual learners learn through seeing and reading. They can recall things that they observe or watch, preferring written instructions, displays, diagrams, films, maps, pictures and demonstrations. Visual learners learn best when:

- in a stimulating and organized environment;
- using diagrams and charts like mind maps, pictures;
- colours highlight important facts or data;
- writing and reading notes.

Auditory learners can listen to and remember verbal information. They learn by discussing and verbalizing ideas. Auditory learners learn best when:

- interviewing, listening to stories and discussions;
- reciting or singing;
- reading aloud or being read to;
- background music is on to help or distract.

Reading and writing learners will be comfortable at university and like to read texts and turn information and data into words. They often spell well and learn from books. Learning this way can be strengthened by:

- using acronyms (such as VARK) to remember facts;
- reading different points of view, noting key points;
- story writing or poetry;
- using sequenced steps to present information.

Kinaesthetic learners benefit from physical experiences, touching, feeling, holding, doing and moving. Spelling and academic writing may not be easy, but learning is increased by:

- playing games involving the body or the senses such as sight, smell, taste, etc.;
- making models or setting up experiments;
- exercising while reflecting on new information;
- acting out situations through role-play.

Try the following Time Out activity to help you apply what you have learnt.

Time Out: Using VARK

Working with a colleague try some of these exercises:
- **make a drink while blindfolded;**
- **go shopping wearing earplugs;**
- **take your colleague shopping in a wheelchair or on crutches;**
- **make a meal while sitting in a wheelchair.**

Reflect on these situations and discuss them with your colleague.
- **What did you learn about having your senses limited like this?**
- **What differences do you think limited sensory perception might have on your work?**

If you are interested in completing an interactive, online questionnaire that will enable you to find out what your VARK learning style is, you can access: http://www. vark-learn.com/english/index.asp.

Deep or surface learning?

Another way to get more out of your learning is to take a 'deep' rather than a 'surface' approach to it. Deep learning involves the critical analysis of new ideas, linking them to already known concepts and principles, and leads to understanding and long-term retention of concepts so that they can be used for problem solving in unfamiliar contexts. Deep learning promotes understanding and application for life. In contrast, surface learning is the tacit acceptance of information and memorization as isolated and unlinked facts. It leads to superficial retention of material for examinations, for example, and does not promote understanding or long-term retention of knowledge and information.

Deep learners are those who:

- aim to make meaning of new knowledge;

- plan and organize study time consistently;

- focus on subject requirements;

- retain more information and do better in the long term.

Adapted from Marton and Säljö (1976, 1997), Entwhistle and Ramsden (1983).

Surface learners tend to accept new knowledge passively, working towards meeting assignment tasks rather than exploring a topic because they are interested in it. For WBL learners, deep learning often comes through undertaking projects linked to work because it is immediately relevant.

You can develop deep study skills by:

- questioning what you are reading, and thinking about its implications;

- linking previous ideas and topics to new knowledge;

- drawing conclusions from reading and considering alternatives in the discussion;

- listing the pros and cons for a discussion;

- planning and organizing study time to ensure it is progressive over time rather than crammed into a few days.

These approaches will promote a deeper understanding of the concepts, theories and applications of learning to a variety of situations or problems experienced at work.

Fatima shares how she valued having a deep approach to her learning on her FD course.

When I was at school I just used to learn everything by rote for the end of year exams but did not really understand in any detail what I had learnt. I could recall facts and figures but was less able to apply detailed theory to analysing complex problems or issues. Since I have undertaken the Foundation Degree I have been able to apply my university learning to my role in the workplace. I have used problem-solving skills, reflection and analysis of best practice evidence to enable me to gain a deeper understanding of what I have learnt.

> *Tools such as learning contracts, reflective diaries, personal development plans and action plans have helped me to apply theory to practice and encouraged me to understand that there are many layers to learning how to solve practical problems and issues. This has, in turn, helped me to move to understanding that I used to just learn about things on a superficial level, never really retaining the important facts and being able to apply these to different situations.*
>
> *Now I have a good understanding of broad concepts that can be applied to a whole range of different settings and scenarios that I come across in the workplace. This in turn has given me self-confidence and the ability to understand the importance of taking responsibility for my actions when I am sound in my own knowledge base. I would never take on aspects of a role that I was not clear or certain about which means that I am in turn a good patient advocate because I know the boundaries and limitations of my own practice.*

The following Time Out activity is designed to help you think about your preferred learning style and your learning habits. Having more insight into your preferences will help you to reflect on whether you need to develop further skills to help you learn and engage with learning in a deeper and more meaningful way. This in turn will help you to identify strategies that you may need to use when undertaking your FD course or learning new skills or roles at work.

Time Out: Considering your preferred learning style.

Consider your learning and personality preferences that you now know.

- **How might this affect your work and learning?**
- **What has been the most important insight so far?**

Now that you have an understanding of your learning style and preferences and the need to take a deep approach to learning, we will consider how learning can happen in your workplace.

What methods of learning occur in the workplace?

There are many ways that learning can happen at work, much of it happens by accident and not all of it is positive. However, four main ways that planned WBL can happen are: *skills-based* learning; *problem-based* learning; *project-based* learning and *social* learning. We will now explore each of these methods in turn.

Skills-based learning

Many practical skills are learnt at work, such as using new equipment or supporting a client's mobility or taking blood. Each workplace will have specific types of practical skills that can only be learnt there. For example, when working in rehabilitation, managing a client's mobility and daily living requirements offer new learning opportunities as these may involve other members of the multi-disciplinary team with specialist skills. Alternatively, an acute care workplace offers skills such as maintaining a client's airway or managing fluid balance. Learning practical skills involves the skill being broken into its component parts to practise each step and perfect it under supervision. Sometimes such skills have to be learnt outside the workplace initially, to ensure that you are safe and are confident when performing in practice, possibly under pressure.

As we explored earlier, activists and pragmatists enjoy learning practical skills, but they may learn poor practice because it seems quicker, which then has to be re-learnt. If you do not feel ready to try things alone for the first time, get your mentor or another colleague to observe your practice. You also need to understand the underpinning theory behind your actions, so ask questions as your skill develops to help remember what is important and why.

Other practical skills include learning how to manage people, or tricky situations or meetings. These 'soft skills' are less easy to get right or wrong, but by observing and listening to more experienced colleagues dealing with situations, you can learn what to do. Try to discuss events afterwards with your mentor to understand why they said or did particular things, so make notes of events to ask them at a convenient point afterwards. These learning activities suit reflectors and auditory learners and are good opportunities to develop these learning styles.

Gathering suitable evidence to demonstrate skills-based learning includes:

- direct or indirect observation by a qualified professional;

- video or audio taping (with the participant's permission);

- **learning diary** or **critical incident record**;

- copy of client records – appropriately anonymized;

- written report from qualified professional;

- designing a poster or information leaflet demonstrating a procedure.

Problem-based learning

Solving work problems can generate both informal and formal learning. An example of informal learning could be helping a client make an informed choice from a range of treatment options and discussing it with them. This requires understanding each option and what it would mean for that particular client's needs, so demonstrating your understanding of available choices by explaining the arguments for and against each one. Formal **problem solving** may be something that a whole team works on, each with different responsibilities for improving or changing practice and may include team meetings, discussions, presentations and literature searches.

Gathering evidence for problem-based learning could include:

- a written summary of options with rational;

- a presentation to colleagues;

- a report used to inform decisions;
- annotated care plans (anonymized and used with permission from your manager);
- learning diary or critical incident extract;
- information leaflets;
- client feedback, either written or recorded (with permission);
- notes of meetings (with permission).

All learning styles can contribute to problem-solving learning. For example, activists may initiate the activity, but the theorists may be the ones who devise the solution, while the pragmatists will implement the best options. Using VARK, visual learners can communicate the plans and outcomes to others through presentations and pictures. Reflectors gather all the information together to summarize the options, and auditory learners can recount the discussions to those who were not able to attend meetings.

Project-based learning

Learning through project work is a valuable tool for WBL as it is usually related to practice. A project may need to be undertaken which involves individuals with different parts of the project in order to solve a work problem, or review, evaluate or introduce new practices. WBL projects can be most motivating when it is your own idea, relating specifically to work that interests you. You will become aware of your role as a worker and learner and it can become difficult to separate out the different roles of learner, worker and researcher. This type of work based research explores what is happening in practice, or what could be done, rather than making a ground-breaking discovery of new knowledge. This is because the project is about a specific context, and is constrained by the work specifications. University requirements for the project will also have to be met, so check these out with your tutor.

Gathering evidence for project-based learning may include:

- a project report;
- project presentation;
- a literature search and/or review;
- case studies or illustrations from practice;
- a product, such as a new policy, procedure, information leaflet, poster;
- learning diary extract.

Undertaking an individual project will extend and develop all learning styles. Your challenge will be to include the styles you find difficult. For example, reflectors may find it difficult to work to a deadline, so set goals and personal deadlines in small chunks to complete it in time. Activists may find it difficult to get down to compiling the report, even though they have completed the practical tasks, so must plan their time and study tasks carefully to complete it. Theorists may get absorbed in the underpinning detail and forget the application to practice, and pragmatists will ensure the project criteria are fulfilled.

Social learning

This is a very powerful way of learning and results from watching others. It includes learning from role-modelling and socialization into work and can be very influential among work teams. A good social learning environment includes:

- strong, affirmative leadership;
- a cohesive work team;
- high practice standards;
- a sound understanding of people;
- a heightened awareness of client needs and rights;
- recognition of staff strengths and potential.

However, not all workplace environments have all these qualities and some may be less positive experiences. A good environment for some learners may be a negative experience for others, but learning does not happen simply by absorbing the working atmosphere. You need to identify learning opportunities for your own needs at work, so consider specific social learning attributes that might be appropriate for you. Examples might include learning to communicate with a client who cannot speak, answering the phone, coaxing a client to drink, or speaking to relatives.

Ideally, identify mentors or colleagues who show particular strengths and learn by asking to shadow them on occasions, or observing how they work. You may watch a professional at your workplace and want them as a mentor because you like their approach, or you may dislike how some staff work and behave, and therefore you decide not to emulate them. Social learning through negative experiences can be powerful too.

Evidence for social learning can include:

- reports from mentors or managers;
- testimonials from clients or colleagues;
- case study examples;
- learning diary extracts;
- letters or emails (with permission).

Most learning styles accommodate social learning approaches, especially those involving observation and listening skills, but extend your knowledge by asking appropriate questions and discussing reasons for professional decisions and actions.

This chapter has introduced you to different learning styles and how you can make the most of your learning in the workplace, by understanding your learning style. In Chapter 4 we will discuss the importance of reflection in WBL.

Key learning points

- Understanding your own preferred learning style will enable you to capitalize on your learning strengths and areas that you need to develop to make the most of future learning opportunities.

- Personal motivation to study and develop is influenced by your personality, personal preferences for learning and your current and future career goals.

- Surface approaches to learning only enable you to hold facts for a short period of time while deeper learning enables you to critique, apply and evaluate new forms of knowledge which will enhance your understanding of workplace problems and enable you to find solutions to improve the quality of care you provide.

- There are four main ways that learning takes place in the workplace: learning practical skills, solving work problems, learning through project work and learning from colleagues.

- Observation and listening skills are important social learning skills that enable you to ask appropriate questions and discuss reasons for professional decisions and actions.

Critical review questions

- **What are the current strengths and limitations of your preferred learning style?**
- **Which of the four main ways of learning in the workplace are your weakest?**
- **What methods can you use to develop these areas further?**

Web links and resources

Higher Education Academy.
http://www.engsc.ac.uk/er/theory/learning.asp

VARK.
http://www.vark-learn.com/english/index.asp

Jung Typology Test.
http://www.humanmetrics.com/cgi-win/JTypes2.asp

Myers and Briggs Personality Type.
http://www.myersbriggs.org/type-use-for-everyday-life/

Reading for interest

Bortherton. G. and Parker, S. (eds) (2010) *Work-based Learning and Practice Placement: A Textbook for Health and Social Care Students*. Newton Abbot: Reflect Press.

Durant, A., Rhodes, G. and Young, D. (2009) *Getting Started with University-level Work Based Learning*. London: Middlesex University Press.

Raelin, J. (2008) *Work-Based Learning: Bridging Knowledge and Action in the Workplace*. Chichester: John Wiley & Sons Ltd.

References

Entwhistle, N.J. and Ramsden, P. (1983) *Understanding Student Learning*. London: Croom Helm.

Honey, P. and Mumford, A. (2006) *The Learning Styles Questionnaire 80-item Version*. Maidenhead: Peter Honey Publications.

Marton, F. and Säljö, R. (1976) On qualitative differences in learning. I, Outcome and process. *British Journal of Educational Psychology*, 46: 4–11.

Marton, F. and Säljö, R. (1997) Approaches to learning, in F. Marton, D.J. Hounsell and N.J Entwhistle (eds) *The Experience of Learning*, 2nd edn. Edinburgh: Scottish Academic Press.

How do you demonstrate learning in the workplace?

4 How does reflection help to support workplace learning?

Mary Northrop

Introduction

In this chapter we demonstrate how reflection enables you to understand workplace and course events as learning incidents. We focus on introducing the concept of reflection and provide an overview of different models of reflection. We introduce some of the skills required to become a reflective practitioner which will be developed further in Chapter 5.

Upon completion of this chapter, you should be able to do the following:

1 Understand the concept of reflection.

2 Identify different models of reflection that promote learning in the workplace.

3 Understand the role that reflection plays in demonstrating evidence of learning in the workplace.

4 Apply different models of reflection to practice.

What is reflection?

Defining reflection

Common descriptions of reflection describe it as the skill of being able to look at situations in order to understand what has been learnt and what future learning needs to occur. Most agree that using reflection increases your self-awareness as a practitioner and this in turn can lead to your development within the workplace.

For example, Boud et al (1985: 19, cited in Ghaye and Lillyman 2006: 7) describes reflection as 'a generic term from those intellectual and effective activities in which individuals engage to explore their experiences in order to lead to a new understanding and appreciation'. The importance here is that reflection is seen as learning from experience (experiential learning) whereby understanding and knowledge are developed through action. This is addressed in more detail in Chapter 2.

The following Time Out activity is designed to help you consider the purpose of using reflection in the workplace.

Time Out: Using reflection in the workplace

Think of an occasion where you found yourself thinking about something you had performed in practice. (This could be a skill you are doing for the first time or interacting with a client or colleague.)

- **What did you focus on?**
- **Why did you think this was important?**
- **What did you learn from thinking about what you did and why?**
- **What knowledge did you realize you already had?**

The situation you choose will differ in terms of what the focus of your reflection was. You may have chosen something practical, or to put into action something you have recently learnt, or develop new ways of working. The important thing is that you tried to identify what went well and what could have been improved. This may have resulted in a range of feelings including being happy with what worked, or feeling anxious with things that did not go well. An important aspect of learning from the situation you have chosen is to consider how a work colleague you respect may deal with this differently. Your workplace mentor might be a suitable role model for you to share this exercise with to find out how they may have handled the situation. This will enable you to highlight gaps in your knowledge or skill base and how you might address these in a supportive environment. Useful questions you might ask to structure this process (Ghaye and Lillyman 2000: 61) include:

- What is my practice like?

- Why is it like this?

- How has it come to be this way?

- What would I like to improve, how and why?

These questions enable you to look at taken-for-granted routines or practices in order to alter care delivery and either improve the quality of your existing practice or develop new practice.

Why would you apply reflection to your practice?

The ability to reflect on practice in the workplace helps you to learn at work for work, and can enhance your ability to solve work based problems and the quality of the care you provide, ensuring a deep approach to your learning. The literature reports the many benefits of using reflection at work. Ghaye and Lillyman (2000: xiv) list 12 principles of reflection that are useful for understanding the contribution that it can make to enhancing your learning and your practice:

1 Reflective practice is about you and your work.

2 Reflective practice is about learning from experience.

3 Reflective practice is about valuing what we do and why we do it.

4 Reflective practice is about learning how to account positively for ourselves and our work.

5 Reflective practice does not separate practice and theory.

6 Reflective practice can help us make sense of our thoughts and actions.

7 Reflective practice generates locally owned knowledge.

8 The reflective conversation is at the heart of the process of reflecting-on-practice.

9 Reflection emphasizes the links between values and actions.

10 Reflection can improve practice.

11 Reflective practitioners develop themselves and their work systematically and rigorously.

12 Reflection involves respecting and working with evidence.

Undertaking the following Time Out activity will enable you to relate this to your practice.

Time Out: How do you apply reflection in your workplace?

Consider the 12 points above in relation to your own practice. Can you think of how you may apply these in your own workplace?

Having discussed the principles of reflection, Taylor (2006) suggests some useful tips for planning and developing reflection skills. Think about these and determine whether any of these tips are useful for your own development. She includes:

- *Taking and making the time to do so by consciously committing to the process and fitting it into an already busy life.* How would you do this?

- *Making the effort by recognizing the value of reflection.* How can you work with your mentor to recognize the role that reflection plays in your learning?

- *Being determined to gain the skills and continue to use them regardless of other commitments or barriers.* What barriers might prevent you from reflecting in the workplace?

- *Having the courage to look at oneself and one's practice and developing solutions which may affect both oneself and others.* How can you develop this confidence and courage?

- *Using humour. Seeing the 'funny side of life' can also be beneficial in changing practice.* When might humour be appropriate and inappropriate?

Having answered these questions, make a note to yourself to revisit your thoughts and feelings at a later date during your FD course. You may choose to use these notes as part of a course assignment or as evidence in your portfolio.

Simon, a first year FD student, explains how he has begun to develop his skills of reflection.

During the first term of the Foundation Degree we were introduced to reflection. This was a word that I had not heard of before but soon realized that this was something which I did in my everyday life but did not consciously engage with this activity. The use of questions to make sense of what I was doing really helped me engage with reflection and to give meaning to my learning.

I chose a really good reflective framework which enabled me to structure my thinking, and I kept a reflective diary to make notes about critical incidents that occurred in the workplace, on aspects of my learning which needed to be further developed, questions to ask my course tutors and workplace mentor, and general notes about links to reading on the course to help me deepen my learning about key concepts. Those notes were invaluable to me during the course as I was able to reflect on the stages of my own personal development as well as rechecking my learning. When it comes to writing the portfolio I will have a range of really useful evidence I can draw upon to demonstrate how I have met the course learning outcomes.

What models and frameworks can you use for reflection?

There are a range of models and frameworks that have been developed and applied across a variety of settings to enable reflection to be a rigorous and structured process. Here we will focus on four approaches:

1 Schön's Theory of Reflection;

2 Kolb's Learning Cycle;

3 Gibb's Reflective Cycle;

4 Driscoll's Developmental Model.

Each approach will be described in turn, with a range of Time Out activities, to enable you to apply them to your practice.

Schön's Theory of Reflection

Schön's (1996) theory of reflection has three main aspects:

* knowing-in-action;
* reflecting-in-action:
* reflection-in-practice.

'Knowing-in-action' is integral to what you do. In order to practise you bring into play what you know and apply this to your actions. The second aspect, 'reflecting-in-action', relates to the ability to think while doing and adapting your own actions to meet the needs of the situation. Schön suggests that this change of action may become part of later practice because if it works you will incorporate this into your repertoire of skills. 'Reflection-in-practice' is explained as looking at the individual's practice as a whole and examining different aspects. Schön suggests that because much of practice is repetitive or similar you can become automatic and 'burnt out'. You see what you expect to see, rather than what is there. By reflecting-in-practice you may be able to recognize where the use of tacit knowledge may be affecting practice and correct this.

Schön suggests reflection-in-practice includes both looking at the situation when it is occurring (reflection in action) and looking back at practice (reflection on action). He also considers that part of reflection includes pre-planning of what you want to reflect on. This is an important consideration when you are undertaking your FD course as you may undertake structured learning activities which ask you to reflect on an aspect of your existing knowledge base or skill set. Undertake the following Time Out activity to help you apply Schön's theory of reflection to a pre-planned aspect of your practice.

Time Out: Pre-planned reflection

Applying Schön's theory of reflection

One of the main functions associated with admission of patients or clients to hospital or to a clinic is that of assessment. Reflect on the last time you completed an assessment and consider the following:

  1 **How did you complete the assessment?**
     a. **Did you use closed or open questions?**
     b. **Who did most of the talking, you or the client?**
     c. **Were there any aspects of the assessment that you completed without asking a question?**
  2 **Is there a different approach you could use and still get the same information?**
  3 **What factors influenced your approach to the documentation?**
     a. **Who are you emulating and why?**
     b. **What is your attitude to completing the assessment?**
     c. **Do you adapt your approach to the needs of the client?**

Next time you complete the assessment form, try changing how you collect the information for one of the aspects being assessed.

  1 **When you changed your approach, how effective was it?**
  2 **Would you incorporate the new approach to your future practice?**
  3 **In completing the exercise, what did you learn about your attitude to completing assessment documentation?**

However, Schön's theory also incorporates unplanned reflection where you adapt within a situation when something unexpected occurs, by reflecting-in-action. Try the following Time Out activity to help you apply this theory to your practice.

Time Out: Reflection-in-action

Think back to an occasion where you changed what you were doing because the situation was not as expected. What was it about the situation that prompted you to adapt what you were doing? What knowledge did you have to enable you to adapt? What was the result?

Schön provides a range of opportunities for reflection and learning in the workplace. As an FD student and/or a practitioner, you bring with you some 'know how' and will be able to apply this to new situations. This knowledge may have been gained from the classroom or your own reading around an issue, or alternatively from observing others (social learning). The concept of social learning is explored in Chapter 3. Knowing-in-action combined with reflection-in-action then allows you to realize when your practice or knowledge base needs changing or adapting. Depending on the task at hand, you may also be supervised, perhaps by a workplace mentor, allowing you to learn from their experience, and this in turn can provide a safety net and sounding board for you to explore your learning needs. As you become more experienced, reflection-in-practice will become integral to your lifelong learning (LLL) and allow you to make informed decisions at the point of care delivery.

Figure 4.1 demonstrates how Schön's theory of reflection can be applied to your practice.

Knowing-in-Action

In the context of the performance of some task, the performer spontaneously initiates a routine of action, which produces an unexpected routine.

↓

Surprise result

The performer notices the unexpected result which he construes as a surprise – an error to be corrected, an anomaly to be made sense of, an opportunity to be exploited.

↓

Knowledge-in-Action

Surprise triggers reflection, directed both to the surprising outcome and to the knowing-in-action that led to it. It is as though the performer asked himself, 'What is this?' and at the same time, 'What understandings and strategies of mine have led me to produce this?'

↓

Reflection-on-Action

The performer restructures his understanding of the situation – his framing of the problem he has been trying to solve, his picture of what is going on, or his strategy of action he has been employing.

↓

Reflection-in Action

On the basis of this restructuring, he invents a new strategy of action.

↓

Reflective practice

He tries out the new action he has invented, running an on the spot experiment whose results he interprets, in turn as a 'solution', an outcome on the wholly satisfactory, or else as a new surprise that calls for a new round of reflection and experimentation.

Figure 4.1 Reflection in Action

Source: Redmond, B. (2006) Reflection in Action. Aldershot: Ashgate Press, p. 37.
Adapted from Schön (1983: 49–69, 1992: 58).
Reproduced with permission from Ashgate Press.

Kolb's Learning Cycle

Kolb's learning cycle (1984) has, as the central focus, the concept of learning through experience and includes reflection as part of this process. It describes four main stages to learning from experience within the workplace: abstract conceptualization; active experimentation; concrete experience and reflective observation. These aspects interlink to form a cycle of learning. The cycle can be repeated to continue the learning process. In order to apply this learning cycle to your own practice we have designed the following Time Out activity so that you can move through each phase of the cycle.

Time Out: Applying Kolb's learning cycle to your workplace

Demonstrating a skill – consider a skill which you need to develop i.e. preparing a trolley for an aseptic procedure and then work through the stages below.

Abstract conceptualization

Part of your learning in the workplace and acquiring new skills will involve you demonstrating your skill development to your mentor. You will need to plan how you will demonstrate that you are competent in your new skill. You will need to show that you understand the evidence base and your organization's policy and procedures; that you are able to safely perform the skill taking into consideration the client's needs; your role and boundaries and that you clearly document your actions.

Active experimentation

This stage of Kolb's cycle involves you designing and planning your demonstration and how you will perform this with your mentor.

Concrete experience

This stage involves you demonstrating your chosen skill to your mentor.

Reflective observation

The reflective observation will incorporate your own reflections and that of your mentor. Consider what went well and what you would change next time you perform your chosen skill. Your mentor may agree with your views and will suggest how your skill performance could be enhanced.

Continuing the cycle

Having worked through the cycle once, you will see that the above example can follow the cycle through again, based on what was decided following the reflective observation.

Gibb's Reflective Cycle

Gibb's (1988) reflective cycle is a well-known cyclical model used for reflection. The model consists of six stages: (1) description, (2) feelings, (3) evaluation, (4) situational analysis, (5) conclusion, and (6) action plan and can be repeated to continue the learning process. Gibb's cycle is designed to relate to a chosen critical learning incident and unlike Kolb, the cycle starts with the description of the event and stops at the action plan. The description of the event allows you to consider factual aspects that place the reflection into context.

The *second stage* enables you to consider your thoughts and feelings. This is where the model differs from others in that it encourages you to address both the factual and subjective aspects of the chosen event.

The *third stage*, evaluation of the event, encourages you to consider areas that went well and those that could be improved and therefore begins the identification of what knowledge or skills you need to develop.

The *fourth stage*, the analysis of the situation, directs you to look at what you know and what you do not know from the chosen incident, but by also examining actions, it enables you to link theory with practice and vice versa, which is an integral part of WBL.

The *fifth stage*, conclusion of what could have been done differently, allows you to consider other strategies which were not used and whether they would have been applicable. The last stage is the formulation of an action plan. This encourages you to consider the way forward, and how the knowledge and skills identified may be applied to your future practice. Gibb's cycle is commonly used in FD courses because it offers a rigorous and structured approach to reflection which helps you to develop the skill of reflection in and on practice. The following Time Out activity will enable you to compare and contrast Kolb's and Gibb's cyclical frameworks and apply these to your own learning needs.

Time Out: Applying Kolb's and Gibb's models to your own learning needs

Both Kolb and Gibb use a cyclical approach in their models. Consider the points below and note down your thoughts:

What are the main differences between the two approaches?

What are the similarities?

What type of learning opportunities do you think will be more appropriate for you to use Kolb's model for reflection?

What type of learning opportunities do you think will be more appropriate for you to use Gibb's model for reflection?

You may have noted that Kolb's cycle can be applied to any learning that occurs in practice, whereas Gibb's model has more of an emotional component and therefore lends itself to complex situations which include examining relationships and ethical aspects of practice. Gibb's model provides more structure than Kolb's cycle, but both emphasize the experience of an event and re-applying the knowledge at a future date. Kolb's and Gibb's models suggest that reflection is cyclical and, like Schön, emphasize the importance of applying learning back into practice and reflecting on its usefulness.

All three models are relevant to your workplace and it is up to you to work with whichever model you feel most comfortable with. This may vary depending on the focus of your reflection. Ask your FD tutors and your workplace mentor to support you in your choice and application of an appropriate model for reflection.

Driscoll's Model of Reflection

John Driscoll's (2007) model of reflection differs from the former models described as it is based on a linear or developmental approach. The model offers trigger questions that enable you to develop your practice and is based on Borton's (1970) education model which uses three developmental questions:

- What?
- So what?
- Now what?

Within these three areas you are encouraged to select the questions you feel are appropriate to your reflection on practice. These are described in Figure 4.2.

1 A description of the event

WHAT? Trigger questions:
- Is the purpose of returning to this situation?
- Happened?
- Did I see/do?
- Was my reaction to it?
- Did other people do who were involved in this?

2 An analysis of the event

SO WHAT? Trigger questions:
- How did I feel at the time of the event?
- Were those feelings I had any different from those of other people who were also involved at the time?
- Are my feelings now, after the event, any different from what I experienced at the time?
- Do I still feel troubled, if so, in what way?
- What were the effects of what I did (or did not do)?
- What positive aspects now emerge for me from the event that happened in practice?
- What have I noticed about my behaviour in practice by taking a more measured look at it?
- What observations does any person helping me to reflect on my practice make of the way I acted at the time?

3 Proposed actions following event

NOW WHAT? Trigger questions:
- What are the implications for me and others in clinical practice based on what I have described and analysed?
- What difference does it make if I choose to do nothing?
- Where can I get more information to face a similar situation again?
- How can I modify my practice if a similar situation was to happen again?
- What help do I need to help me 'action' the results of my reflection?
- Which aspect should be tackled first?
- How will I notice that I am any different in clinical practice?
- What is the main learning that I take from reflecting on my practice in this way?

Figure 4.2 Driscoll's model of reflection
Source: Driscoll (2007: 44).

The first of the three questions, 'What?, enables you to consider the context in which reflection is taking place. It asks you to describe the situation and within that situation what is being reflected on. By providing a description of the event, either verbally or by writing things down, you may see different perspectives, or clarify the issue that you wish to reflect on.

The 'So What?' begins the analysis of the event. It enables you to try and make sense of the situation in relation to your own learning both emotionally and practically. It allows you to explore your perceptions of the event and whether they are similar to others involved. It will also enable you to reflect on any changes that are necessary in your own practice, either through changing your attitude or values, or by highlighting gaps in your knowledge or skills base.

The 'Now What?' aspect of the model follows on from the analysis and leads to new learning or applying what you have learnt back to the same or a similar situation. The following Time Out activity will help you to find a suitable model of reflection that will work for you.

Time Out: Finding a reflective model that works for you!

The previous section has outlined a range of models and frameworks for reflecting on learning in the workplace. From the models provided consider:

- **Which model/framework do you prefer and why?**
- **Which model/framework do you think you are less likely to use and why?**
- **Do any of the models/frameworks relate to how you have used reflection in the past?**

Your choice of model may be influenced by the amount of structure you need in order to reflect effectively. Some of you will prefer a broader approach such as Schön, where you decide what to ask. Others will prefer a more comprehensive list of questions, for example, those provided by Driscoll. For some of you, flexibility is more important and you may develop experience in using a range of models/frameworks. More detailed examples of how to apply Driscoll's and Gibb's models are provided in Chapter 5. After reading Chapter 5 you may like to review the exercise above and see if your initial thoughts have changed.

Fatima, an FD graduate student reflects on her experiences of using a range of different models.

When I began to formalize my reflection on my Foundation Degree, I chose Gibb's model as I liked the structure it provided. This is because I was not really used to thinking in a structured way and lacked the confidence to reflect on my own. However, as I became more confident during the course I began to experiment with a range of different models.

I found that I liked Driscoll's model because it was less formal than Gibb's and gave me more chance to develop my skills of reflection. Our action learning set enabled me to understand that my peers have different preferences and needs when choosing a model of reflection. The most important thing is that you should choose one that suits you. This may vary as you gain confidence in your ability to reflect in and on action and at different stages of your learning. My peers helped me enormously to understand how we all have different styles and preferences. The essential thing is that there is no 'one size fits all' approach. Choose what suits you best and works well for you.

How do you demonstrate reflection in your Foundation Degree course?

In Chapter 1, Tom Aird talks about the importance of your FD course helping you to identify your learning needs, developing learning opportunities to enhance your knowledge base, and recording your learning through a range of structured activities. Your FD course will enable you to focus on specific aspects of WBL and to aid your decision-making in relation to answering the questions: *What do I need to learn?, What do I already know?* and *How can I incorporate this in to my future work?*

For example, one of the assignments for your FD course might include discussing a **case study** and how you would implement change to practice in your clinical area. Consider the following case study example:

Case study

An FD student employed as a Health Care Assistant in a district nursing team regularly visits care homes to undertake leg ulcer dressings which have been prescribed by a registered professional. While doing so she notes that one client's legs are not being washed. She has learnt that this will impair wound healing (*learning identified*). She initially examines the evidence-base that underpins recommended care guidelines for leg ulcers (*learning added*), and then discusses this with her mentor and one of the care home managers. The result of this reflection is the development of a training programme as part of her FD assessment (*learning recognized*) for care home staff. This training programme provides best practice guidelines for leg ulcer care and is now being implemented in other care homes in the area. For this project she received a distinction in her FD course and an award for outstanding practice achievement.

Jasper (2006) provides criteria for selecting a reflective framework which also acts as a checklist in relation to what you want to reflect on, how you wish to reflect and the purpose of reflection. These criteria may be useful in your FD course and you can see the framework in Figure 4.3.

What am I trying to achieve?

- My own learning or identification of my learning needs
- Increased understanding
- To take a different perspective on an experience or event
- Practice development

How do I want to reflect?

- In my head
- Verbally: in a dialogue, in a group, with facilitation
- In writing

Who do I want to reflect with?

- Myself
- One other person
- Other colleagues/students
- My supervisor/academic tutor
- Another group of people

What sort of structure do I want to use?

- Broad questions
- Specific questions
- A reflective cycle
- A framework that leads me towards action
- A framework that leads me towards a deeper understanding
- A facilitative and developmental framework

When do I want to reflect?

- Immediately
- After I get home from work
- During the next session at university
- During **clinical supervision**
- At some other convenient time

Where do I want to reflect?

- Within the clinical environment
- At home
- At university
- In a quiet area away from the clinical environment
- In a neutral place

What are the values underpinning and inherent to the model?

- How do these fit with my own values as a practitioner?

Figure 4.3 Criteria for selecting a reflective framework
Source: Jasper (2006: 62).

The following Time Out activity enables you to apply these criteria to your FD course.

> **Time Out: Using Jasper's criteria to select an appropriate reflective framework**
>
> An important part of WBL is to understand what you need to achieve in order to meet the learning outcomes for your FD course. Looking at one of your course's learning outcomes, identify an aspect of practice that you wish to reflect on. Use Jasper's criteria above in Figure 4.3, decide how you are going to carry out the reflection and why.

Developing new knowledge through reflection

Your FD course will encourage you to reflect on different types of knowledge. This is likely to include:

- *Scientific knowledge* – the evidence base which underpins your practice. Examples include national benchmark standards, National Institute Clinical Excellence (NICE) guidelines, research evidence, quality measures, policies and procedures.

- *Personal knowledge* – knowledge you have gained through experience, some of which you may not be aware of. This type of knowledge comes from your life experiences in general and interaction with those around you as well as your interests and passions. This is also known as **tacit knowledge**.

- *Practical/aesthetic knowledge* – understanding how you do things in practice and includes interpersonal skills. The use of touch, verbal and non-verbal communication skills helps you to demonstrate empathy and to build a relationship with the clients and their families within your care.

- *Traditional knowledge* – the way in which things have always been done in practice.

- *Knowledge from authority* – this can include policies, procedures and evidence based guidelines or national standards.

- *Trial and error* – experimenting until you find what works.

- *Role modelling* – emulating someone else who you respect and adapting your practice to include their ways of working/thinking/behaving in practice.

- *Ethical knowledge* – understanding right from wrong and applying professional values and attitudes to your practice. This might include, for example, understanding the legal aspects of drug administration or safeguarding vulnerable adults. It includes your duty of care, responsibility and accountability to abide by professional codes of conduct and maintain confidentiality.

(Ghaye and Lillyman (2000).

Try the following Time Out activity to help you think about the types of knowledge you use in your workplace practice.

> **Time Out: What knowledge do you use in the workplace?**
>
> **Looking at an aspect of your workplace duties, write down the different types of knowledge which you drew on to carry out the task/skill.**

You might find that you have used all of the types of knowledge we have referred to in this Time Out activity but you were unaware of this. Reflection therefore enables you to gain a better understanding of the types of knowledge you apply to your workplace practice.

This chapter has introduced different models and frameworks for reflection which you could use on your FD or in the workplace. In Chapter 5 we will discuss how you may use a range of different strategies and tools to help you develop as a reflective learner.

Key learning points

- Reflection will support a deep approach to learning as it allows you to consider a situation and identify what you have learnt and any further learning needs.

- The model or framework you choose is personal and may be influenced by the context of the event you are reflecting on.

- Jasper (2006) provides criteria for selecting a reflective framework which also acts as a checklist to ensure effective reflection on practice.

- Reflection enables you to explore a range of knowledge which may be required in your workplace, including scientific, personal, practical and trial and error.

> **Critical review questions**
> - **Which model or framework of reflection suits your learning style?**
> - **How can reflection enhance your workplace role?**
> - **What new knowledge have you developed as a result of reflection?**

Reading for interest

Driscoll, J. (ed.) (2007) *Practising Clinical Supervision: A Reflective Approach for Healthcare Professionals*, 2nd edn. Edinburgh: Baillière Tindall.

Ghaye, T. and Lillyman, S. (2000) *Reflection: Principles and Practice for Healthcare Professionals*. Dinton: Quay Books.

Ghaye, T. and Lillyman, S. (2006) *Learning Journals and Critical Incidents*, 2nd edn. London: Quay Books.

Gibb, G. (1988) *Learning by Doing: A Guide to Teaching and Learning Methods*. Oxford: Further Education Unit.

References

Borton, T. (1970) Reach, Teach & Touch. London: McGraw Hill.

Boud, D., Keough, R. and Walker, D. (1985) *Reflection: Turning Experience into Learning*. London, Kogan Page, cited in T. Ghaye and S. Lillyman (2006) *Learning Journals and Critical Incidents*, 2nd edn. London: Quay Books.

Driscoll, J. (ed.) (2007) *Practising Clinical Supervision: A Reflective Approach for Healthcare Professionals*, 2nd edn. Edinburgh: Baillière Tindall.

Ghaye, T. and Lillyman, S. (2000) *Reflection: Principles and Practice for Healthcare Professionals*. Dinton: Quay Books.

Ghaye, T. and Lillyman, S. (2006) *Learning Journals and Critical Incidents*, 2nd edn. London: Quay Books.

Gibb, G. (1988) *Learning by Doing: A Guide to Teaching and Learning Methods*. Oxford: Further Education Unit.

Jasper, M. (2006) *Professional Development, Reflection, and Decision Making*. Oxford: Blackwell.

Johns, C. and Freshwater, D. (eds) (2005) *Transforming Nursing through Reflective Practice*, 2nd edn. Oxford: Blackwell Publishing.

Kolb, D. (1984) *Experiential Learning: Experience as the Source of Learning and Development*. Englewood Cliffs, NJ: Prentice-Hall.

Redmond, B. (2006) *Reflection in Action*. Aldershot: Ashgate Press.

Schön, D. (1996) *The Reflective Practitioner: How Professionals Think in Action*. Aldershot: Arena Ashgate Publishing Ltd.

Taylor, B. (2006) *Reflective Practice: A Guide for Nurses and Midwives*, 2nd edn. Maidenhead: Open University Press.

How do you develop as a reflective learner?

Jayne Crow

Introduction

Reflection is a method by which experience may be turned into learning, and in Chapter 4 you were introduced to this concept and some examples of models of reflection. Reflection is a skill and as such needs to be practised and developed if you are to maximize your learning. This chapter will build on reflective theory and will present a variety of strategies and tools to help you reflect effectively, whether you choose to do so alone or with others. It will focus particularly on the process of reflecting 'in action' and 'on action'. In many cases extracts of reflective writing will be used to illustrate how you might apply theory to practice. The learning styles discussed in Chapter 3 identify the importance of a 'reflective' learner as someone who likes to think about things in detail before they take action. It is the nature of this thoughtful approach and how to evidence this which will be discussed in this chapter. If you are naturally a reflective learner, you will find the activities attractive. If not, the activities may take more practice and perseverance to master. It is worth taking time to do this because learning through reflection is a key tool for life long learning (LLL).

Upon completion of this chapter, you should be able to do the following:

1 **Apply reflective theory to practice to promote work based learning.**

2 **Develop reflection skills to promote life-long learning.**

3 **Understand how a range of evidence can be presented to demonstrate reflection in and on action in the workplace.**

When is reflection 'in action' and 'on action' appropriate?

Reflection 'in action' usually takes the form of thinking something through while in the situation. It may or may not involve a brief discussion with a colleague or mentor at the time. Conversely, reflection 'on action' takes place after the event. Reflection 'in action' may be an end in itself but it can also be followed up later by further reflection ('on action'). It may be useful to employ a strategy to prompt the revisiting of a situation to enable more learning to take place. Ghaye & Lillyman (2006) recommends making notes while at work to record details of 'reflection in action' at the time of the episode. You may find it useful to carry a reflective diary or journal with you to enable you to make a note of your thoughts, feelings or key questions that arise from your practice. The following Case Study presents an excerpt from a reflective diary and is designed to help you to think about how you could use this in your own practice.

> **Case Study: An example from a reflective diary**
>
> *What?*
>
> Clients in a GP waiting room were upset and frightened by the aggressive behaviour of a fellow client who was queuing at reception and complaining about a late appointment.
>
> *When?*
>
> **Mon, 24 August 2010, 10am**
>
> *Reflection*
>
> I feel helpless. I questioned whether the aggressive behaviour of the client could have been predicted or avoided and whether the distressed behaviour of the clients in the waiting room could have been handled differently.
>
> *Action*
>
> I made time to talk to the other clients in the waiting room but I found it difficult to reassure them. I need to explore this further in terms of my own learning. I plan therefore to use this reflection diary to discuss with my mentor on Friday, 28 August 2010.

The above case study shows how you can make important notes about a situation as they occur and you can use these notes to discuss with your course tutor or mentor. In this way you can demonstrate reflection on action and explore opportunities for learning and improving practice. It allows the situation to be explored and analysed in depth using a structured reflective cycle that enables you to make sense of your practice. You may go on to look in more detail about what you did, how you felt, what information you drew on or needed to access. You may, for instance, identify that you need to find out more about the policy and procedure implemented in these situations. Does it take clients' safety and feelings into account, for example? You may make plans to instigate discussion at a team meeting on managing aggressive behaviour. Having the brief notes recorded at the time is a useful way of evidencing reflection 'in action' that can then be followed with the written account of your reflection 'on action'.

Reflecting 'on action' may take place at any time after the event such as directly at the end of a shift or after a few days. However, it may also be useful to reflect on practice that took place a while ago (as long as you can remember the details of what happened). This is often revealing, in that looking back on our thoughts and actions across time can show how our thoughts, knowledge, attitudes and/or practice have developed, or the ways in which past experiences have influenced current thinking and practice. Your FD course is likely to encourage you to use a **reflective diary** or **journal** as a structured learning process, and your assignments or portfolio may encourage you to use excerpts from your diary to demonstrate achievement of your course learning outcomes. The following Time Out activity will enable you to reflect on your own personal and professional development during your FD course.

Time Out: Reflection on your FD course experiences

If you have been on your present FD course for some time, take a moment to reflect back on your experience of the first day of the course. Compare your thoughts and feelings then with your thoughts and feelings now. Are they different? If so, how and why? What have you learned since that time?

Fatima explains how she developed her reflection skills to moving beyond reflecting on action to reflecting in action.

When I started my FD course I used a range of searching skills to find out more information to help me reflect on what had happened at work or in the classroom as I analysed significant learning events in my development. This reflection was always structured and took place AFTER the event. Now that I have completed the course and am working as a Band 4 Assistant Practitioner, I find that I am questioning my practice and that of others as a natural part of my daily work to ensure that we are providing the best quality of evidence-based service. Because I am more confident in my skills and abilities I find that I am reflecting action as situations occur in order to make judgements about how to solve problems or provide the best outcome for clients in my care. This is a significant shift in the way in which I think and behave.

What tools can you use to develop your reflection skills?

Chapter 4 explored models and frameworks to promote reflection. These had a common theme of action, description, reflection and on to further action. We identified that no one model is right or comprehensive, they all have their strengths. However, we presented Jasper's (2006) criteria for making an informed choice about which model of reflection is right for you (see fig.4.3). Most importantly the aim is to instill in you a habit of reflection that lasts beyond your FD course and provides a method of learning for your whole professional life.

We will now turn our attention to a range of tools and strategies that will help you to develop your reflective skills. The first of these is **critical incident analysis**.

Critical incident analysis

The term 'critical' can be applied to a variety of incidents. The most important factor here is that it is meaningful, poses questions about your practice and represents a significant learning opportunity. Examples of critical incidents might be:

- an incident that is an ordinary experience;
- an incident where the experience did not go to plan (these may be positive as well as negative experiences);
- an incident that went well;
- an incident that reflects the values and beliefs held by the individual;
- an incident that identifies the contribution of qualified practitioners;
- an incident that allows the identification of learning.

As you can see from these examples, it is the individual who decides whether an incident is significant or not. It does not have to be extraordinary, dangerous or an emergency. In order to analyse a critical incident in a structured way, it is possible to apply both Gibb's and Driscoll's models of reflection as demonstrated in the following examples. Try the following Time Out activity to help you apply these models.

Time Out: Using Gibb's reflective cycle

- **Read the worked example below. It shows how a practitioner used Gibb's reflective cycle to reflect on an experience at work.**
- **Once you have read it, choose an experience from your own practice and write about it using the same headings.**
- **Then ask yourself, has the process of writing about the experience made you think in more detail about it? Were you surprised about anything that you remembered doing or feeling? Have you learnt anything from writing your reflection down? Was Gibb's model useful in focusing your thoughts? How might it benefit your learning to share your piece of writing with someone else?**

Examine the following case study which demonstrates how Gibb's reflective cycle was used to support reflection-on-action.

Case Study: Visiting Mr Khan

Description

What happened?

I visited Mr Khan who lives alone and has a terminal illness. During our conversation he told me he was frightened of dying alone. It took me by surprise so I said, 'That's natural, I suppose. Perhaps it is best not to think along those lines as it will only get you down.' I told him that I would inform the community nurse about what he had said so that she could help. I found this difficult to talk about so I changed the subject to a more upbeat one and he didn't say any more about it. I completed my visit and left as soon as possible.

Feelings

What were you thinking and feeling?

I was taken completely by surprise by the subject of dying. I felt so sorry for him and just wished I could fix the situation but knew I could not. I wanted to make things better for him but I felt embarrassed and inadequate because I did not know what to say and I did not want to make things worse so I said something that I hoped was comforting and practical. I was relieved to leave but then felt guilty and sad.

Evaluation

What was good and bad about the experience?

I suppose it was good that he felt able to talk to me about dying. He must have felt he could trust me. I think I should report this experience to my manager so that a referral to the Macmillan Nursing Services can be made. This will allow him to gain the expert support which he needs. However, it made me realize I need to improve my knowledge of how to communicate effectively with patients who are dying and to listen to their needs even if I do not have the solutions at the time.

Analysis

What sense can you make of the situation?

Mr Khan had opened up to me about his feelings about dying alone. He had bravely indicated that he wanted to talk to me about this. I panicked and felt too embarrassed to let him continue so I responded immediately to try and fix the situation by saying I would 'solve' 'the problem' by bringing in someone else to deal with it. I thereby communicated to Mr Khan both verbally and non-verbally that I did not want to have this conversation with him, and he responded by going along with the change of subject. I realized that I behaved in this manner because I do not have the experience of working with dying patients and I have not had the opportunity to develop an understanding of the sorts of questions and issues that dying patients might present. I also realize that the power of non-verbal communication is influential when dealing with difficult issues.

Conclusion

What else could you have done?

I could have listened to Mr Khan and taken the time to enable him to identify and explore the issues and questions that he had. Even if I was not able to answer these questions myself, we could have formed a list of questions together that I could then use to discuss further with more appropriately qualified colleagues. By sitting with him, making good eye contact and conveying a relaxed body posture I could have indicated that I was paying full attention to what he was saying and was willing to listen.

Action Plan

If it arose again what would you do?

- *Explore with my mentor and course tutor how to improve verbal and non-verbal communication skills.*

- *Seek guidance from the literature to enhance my knowledge and understanding of terminal illness, death and dying.*
- *Explore with fellow students what works well for them and what does not work so well and why.*
- *Talk to a local chaplain about how to support people with terminal illness and deal with death and dying.*
- *Seek out opportunities to work a couple of shifts in a palliative care setting.*

Following on from this, we present a critical incident analysis using Driscoll's model of structured reflection. Have a go at completing the following Time Out activity.

Time Out: Using Driscoll's (2007) model of structured reflection

- **Read the worked example below. It shows how a practitioner has used Driscoll's model of structured reflection to reflect on an experience at work.**
- **Once you have read it, choose an experience from your own practice and write about it under the same headings.**
- **Then ask yourself, has the process of writing about the experience made you think in more detail about it? Were you surprised about anything that you remembered doing or feeling? Have you learned anything from writing your reflection down? Was Driscoll's model useful in focusing your thoughts? How might it benefit your learning to share your piece of writing with someone else?**

Below is another case study example demonstrating a structured reflection using Driscoll's model of reflection.

Case Study: Grace

What?

As a FD student I was asked by one of the Sisters in my team to visit Grace in her home and to take a photograph of her wound as she 'likes to see how it is doing'.

I had not visited Grace before and when I arrived at her front door I was surprised that it was opened by a lady in a wheelchair. She had only one leg. I learned that her other leg had been amputated below the knee three years ago. She later told me that the problem was related to her diabetes and had begun with an infected toe. I read from her medical history that she had ischaemic heart disease and poor circulation.

Grace greeted me and as we had not met before, she asked if I was new. I replied that I had only been with the team for a few months and had been asked to photograph her wound. This pleased her as she said it had not been photographed for some time.

Whilst Grace proceeded to roll up her trouser leg I was reading the care plan to establish what care I was to give. The care plan listed all the dressings and care to be carried out. On inspection of Grace's leg it appeared to be heavily bandaged and demonstrated considerable seepage which concerned me. I was mildly relieved that the bandages were not compression bandages as these are not appropriate for the treatment of arterial ulcers. I quickly realized that I did not have sufficient knowledge or training in what appeared to be advanced wound care management and I informed Grace that I should call one of the qualified staff to deal with this. Grace replied that she knew exactly how the wound should be dressed and that she could talk me through it. I stated that I did not wish to exacerbate the condition of the wound through my lack of knowledge and I went to telephone my colleagues on shift but received no reply. On returning, I found that Grace had already removed her wound dressings and positioned herself for me to photograph the wound. She seemed quite intent on having the photographs taken and totally unconcerned that I was inexperienced in this type of wound care. She appeared confident that we could successfully tend the wound. I was struck by how brave and determined she was. Following Grace's instruction I cleansed and dressed the wound. I documented what I had done and left. On my return to the office I reported what had happened to my team leader.

So what?

My immediate concern on seeing the seepage on Grace's bandage was the potential risk of infection and further injury to her if I removed them. Grace then took the decision out of my hands by taking down the dressing herself. Once she had exposed the wound I became more anxious as I realized that the ulcers were leaking considerably.

I felt angry that I had been placed in a position in providing care for a client whose needs exceeded my wound care abilities. I felt unsupported as there was no-one at the other end of the telephone whom I could ask for advice. I felt it was unfair to put both myself and Grace at risk.

Having completed the wound dressing, Grace thanked me very much for all I had done and remarked again that she had no problem with me coming to dress the wound again. However, I did not feel the same way and decided that until I gained more knowledge of wound care and improved technique I would decline to visit patients who require advanced wound care. I still feel that. Since that time I have thought about the incident a lot because I found it so disturbing and maintain my view that I should not have been put in that situation.

In retrospect and on a more positive note I did dress the wound satisfactorily and was thus able to protect it from further injury or infection. Thanks to this incident with Grace, I now have more confidence in my ability to keep outwardly calm, think on my feet and rise to the occasion in an emergency.

Now what?

There are legal issues of accountability and responsibility linked to this case as I did not want to cause Grace harm through my lack of knowledge and training in advanced wound care. I have referred to our Trust policy and literature on this subject and have pointed out to the qualified staff in the team the implications for both parties of my being placed in a situation requiring me to attempt care that I consider at the limits or beyond my abilities.

I was placed in a situation where 'doing nothing' was no longer an option as far as I was concerned because of the infection risk. I had tried to get help and advice but had failed to get a response. I felt the safest thing to do was to dress the wound as documented and advise the trained staff as soon as possible. This is one of those situations where one has to choose the action leading to least harm. I do not regret my decision but do regret finding myself in such a position.

The main things I have learnt from this experience and the first thing that I will action is to take steps to prevent myself being placed in such a position again. I intend to question my allocation of wound care patients to ascertain the extent of their wounds, and either to decline what is outside my capabilities, or preferably request that a qualified member of staff accompanies me. However, should I find myself in this position again, I would be forced to take the matter to my Matron, as the whole ethos of patient care is 'best practice' carried out by competent staff.

I have realized that I need to gain more understanding of and skills in wound care and will try to engage the qualified staff in facilitating my development in this area as much as possible. I will volunteer to observe and assist qualified staff in dressing slightly more advanced wounds. I will also apply to undertake a wound management course. Nevertheless until I receive the appropriate training, I shall remain working within my scope of practice.

An unexpected result of this incident is that I have learnt that patients can be expert teachers and knowledgeable in their own care.

We have presented case study examples of two of the models of reflection that are available to guide you. You may wish to use some of the other models described in Chapter 4 to structure your own reflective writing. Both case studies demonstrate reflection in and on action.

What other tools are available to support your reflection?

As we have noted, critical incident analysis is a popular vehicle for reflection but it is by no means the only strategy to help you learn and improve your practice. Here we present a range of strategies you may like to use as catalysts for reflection.

Time Out: Activities

Activity 1 Observation exercise

Take half an hour to act as an observer in your work environment. Just sit and watch the reception desk area or a waiting area or interactions during a consultation. Try to see the environment with new eyes in the way that a newcomer sees it. Write up your reflection on the experience.

Activity 2 Reflecting on communication skills

Attend a meeting at work and rather than participate, just observe the communication that takes place. Look out particularly for non-verbal cues and responses. Reflect on how the communication skills of the participants facilitated or disrupted good communication. Write up your reflection on what you see and hear.

Activity 3 Using the media as a stimulus to reflection on your work

Watch or listen to relevant broadcasts e.g.:

- **Film, TV and radio** – fiction/dramas relating to the experiences of service-users.
- **Documentaries and news stories,** e.g. about abuse in care, care rationing, health scares, etc.
- **Broadcast interviews with service users.**

Consider how the item has influenced your knowledge, way of thinking or your attitudes/assumptions. How did it make you feel? Why? Has it highlighted any gap in your knowledge that you need to address? Will it influence your behaviour, your approach to your work, your motivation, and your intentions for the future? Write up your reflection.

Reflective writing

A further way of developing your ability to reflect in and on practice is through **reflective writing**. There is a strong argument that limiting yourself to **analytical writing** (trying to make sense of the situation) in reflection is counterproductive and that using your imagination and creativity can also promote learning and improve practice (Winter et al. 1999). This could take a variety of forms. For example, you could write:

- an imagined account of the experience of a service user receiving your care;

- a poem;

- a fictional letter written by an angry service user or carer.

Most people have not written in this way since their early teens but if you have a go you may surprise yourself and the process can be very enjoyable and cathartic as well as revealing and informative to practice. Below we present an example of **empathetic writing**.

An imagined account written from the perspective of a service user

I feel really uncomfortable. I felt so good when the carers settled me down in this position; all cosy and warm in my bed, just like a bird in a nest. I even drifted off into a little sleep and goodness knows I need to get some sleep. The noise in this ward is unbelievable, all crashing and banging and buzzing and bleeping. I feel exhausted and I seem to have been awake for days on end being pulled about and 'investigated', hauled out of bed, into chairs, back into bed, poked, prodded, questioned. They have to do it, of course; I understand that.

What is the time, I wonder? If I can just move my head enough I might be able to see that clock on the opposite wall. That can't be right, can it? Is it really only 15 minutes since they settled me down? I felt so comfortable but now my arm has gone to sleep as I am lying on it and there seems to be something digging into my shoulder – it is beginning to really hurt and now to cap it all I need to go to the toilet. Surely I don't need to go just yet; I can't bear the thought of being hoisted up again. I just want to get into a comfortable position and go off to sleep; I am so, so tired. I never thought I would give anything and everything to be able to turn over in bed on my own! How we take such precious things for granted.

I'll try to put off calling them. Maybe I can hold on for a bit longer. They are really busy and I don't want to be a bother. I heard them talking about another patient on the ward saying how demanding she is and that she is 'heavy'. I wonder what they say about me. I wonder if they call me 'heavy'. I don't want them to think of me like that. I depend on them so much and I really don't want to make them cross. I'll wait a bit longer.

Surely it is more than 5 minutes since I looked at that clock. I seem to have been lying here in pain for ages and I'm absolutely busting to go to the toilet now. I can hardly feel my arm apart from a throbbing feeling and I wonder if this thing, whatever it is, that is digging in my shoulder is damaging my skin; Maybe I'll get a sore like the one my neighbour got in hospital. It never really healed. Oh God, I'm going to have to ring the bell and ask them to help me again. Please don't let them be angry with me and please don't let me wet the bed before they come.

Having read this example, undertake the following Time Out activity.

Time Out: Empathetic imaginative writing

- **Read the imagined account in the example above. What did you learn from reading this account?**
- **Now choose a service user that you have encountered in your practice and try to put yourself in their shoes and write an imagined account of their experience of the service you provide. Try particularly to convey what you imagine their thoughts and feelings are rather than just describing what happens to them. Try to write using the language they would use and focus on their concerns.**
- **How did it feel to write this piece? What have you learned from writing empathetically? Does this writing highlight any areas of your practice that are helpful or less helpful to the service user? Is there anything that you can do to improve their experience by modifying your practice or changing a system?**

Of course we can never really know how another person feels, but writing in this way will help you develop and evidence your empathetic skills as you try to put yourself in the situation of another human being, and to see the world through their eyes.

Sharing and discussing such accounts can refocus you and your team on the importance of individualizing care and prioritizing dignity and respect in your practice. Your FD course should provide you with an opportunity to engage in discussion with fellow students to explore this kind of activity and you can also share this in the workplace with your mentor or other colleagues. One of the key skills that reflective writing can help you to develop is self-awareness.

Developing self-awareness in reflective writing

An important part of reflection is learning to question yourself in order to develop your self-awareness. It involves looking at your own interpretations of events and examining how your assumptions, values and beliefs influence your reactions and actions. Subconsciouly you carry all sorts of baggage from your past experience (both personal and professional), and it is important that you recognize how this influences your behaviour, and the decisions you make. It is important for you to understand that you never go into any situation with a mind like a 'blank slate'. The act of thinking about your own values, beliefs and assumptions, and becoming aware of these is known as **reflexivity**. Reflexivity then, is an important part of reflection on action because as a novice you will be encouraged to explore your values and beliefs as part of your FD course, either through action learning or using structured models of reflection. Expert practitioners tend to have a high degree of self-awareness and are therefore able to suspend their values and beliefs when dealing with difficult situations. In other words they are aware of their values and beliefs while they are reflecting in action. This enables them to avoid stereotyping or prejudging situations, people or events because they are aware of their own feelings, thoughts and values and how these can influence their behaviour and actions. The following Time Out will help you consider your own values, beliefs and assumptions.

Time Out: Developing your self-awareness

- **Read the journal diary entry below.**
- **You can see that the practitioner's values, beliefs and personal experience influenced her practice. Through her reflective diary and the process of reflecting on her actions she has been able to explore how these have influenced her professional practice and judgements made in the care for the client concerned.**
- **Think about a recent care episode which was influenced by your own values, beliefs and assumptions. Make a note in your reflective diary of these values and beliefs and how they influence your practice.**
- **Discuss with your mentor how your values and beliefs differ from theirs, whether there are any similarities or overlaps. Then identify a recent care episode that you were both involved in that you can explore together. Reflect on your values, beliefs and assumptions and how these influenced your behaviour, actions and care outcomes.**

The following case study helps you to see how becoming aware of your values and beliefs can enable you to overcome subconscious prejudices in your practice. Through the use of a reflective diary, it is possible to analyse how your behaviours and actions might be developed and improved and how new learning can take place as a result of becoming more self-aware.

Case Study: Maria

I visit an elderly client, Maria, in her own home on a routine call and she tells me she has not seen anyone else since my colleague visited her last week. Her son lives in the next village but has not visited for six months. I show my disapproval of his behaviour by the way that I respond and suggest very strongly that the client telephones her son to tell him of her situation and ask him to visit.

Later I make a note in my reflective diary:

> *'I felt really angry when Maria said her son had not been "near nor by" for so long. How can he be so uncaring when she is so vulnerable? A little bit of help from him would make the world of difference to her'.*

Reflexive analysis

Looking at my reaction more closely I can see that I react very protectively and am maternalistic towards Maria and thinking about this further, to elderly clients in general. I think this is because I am reminded of my own grandmother who was very dear to me and who was very frail in her last years of life.

I feel strongly that families have a 'duty' to care for their elderly relatives in need. Doing one's duty is important in my view. I felt angry with her son and I am sure this came across in my tone and she saw that I thought he should help more. On reflection I let my personal views influence my practice too much. I should try to stop myself making judgements on the basis of so little information. For example I know nothing of the history of Maria's relationship with her son, or what his situation is currently. I certainly shouldn't have let my views come across so strongly.

Using reflective writing as a tool to develop your self-awareness is an important part of your ongoing development. However, there are often challenges associated with how much information to reveal, especially when your writing may be part of a structured FD course assessment, because you have a duty to protect your client's identity and respect confidentiality.

Honesty and confidentiality in reflective writing

When you write down your reflections in a diary, log or a course assignment there will always be a question as to how honestly and comprehensively you write. You certainly need to be honest with yourself if you are to grow in self-awareness and learn from your experience. However, you will also be aware that what is written may be seen by others. It is important therefore to be clear about who will see the written text and that you need to protect the confidentiality of those individuals and organizations that you are writing about.

Reflective writing for assignments

If you are writing reflectively for an assignment, it is likely that your course assignments will have guidelines for you to follow with regard to anonymity and confidentiality, and will make it clear who will normally have access to the script. (This will usually be the teaching and administrative team on the course and the external assessor.) It would be usual in these circumstances to anonymize names, organizations and locations and to take steps to protect the identity. If unsafe practice is identified in your assignment, then the course tutor will have a duty to act on that information. This would normally be done in collaboration with you. Your course tutors have a duty of care and responsibility to protect the general public and to report unsafe practice wherever it is identified. This might take the form of your course tutor having to contact the practice area concerned to discuss the reported unsafe practice further. The university or workplace will have policies and procedures for dealing with these circumstances when they arise.

Reflective journals and confidentiality

Your reflective journal or diary is personal to you and the notes that you keep to help you to reflect in and on action will differ from those of other students and colleagues. What you must bear in mind is that the entries you make should promote confidentiality at all times because you may choose to use extracts from your diaries in your course assignments or through action learning discussion groups. Sometimes students choose to use excerpts from their diaries in a course assignment to illustrate structured reflection on a case study. This is a good idea because it enables you to reflect on your actions and the thoughts, feelings and experiences of your clients and your colleagues who may have been involved in a critical incident with you. Another occasion where it may be appropriate to utilize extracts from your diary would be in the presentation of a course portfolio. Portfolios often enable you to demonstrate integration of your learning and reflections on your learning progress and career development and can use a range of evidence to support course learning outcomes.

Reflecting alone or with others?

You may choose to reflect with mentors/colleagues, your manager, in groups, pairs or alone. There is no single right or wrong way. It all depends on the context, feasibility, purpose and personal preference. Table 5.1 summarizes the advantages and disadvantages of reflecting alone and with others.

Table 5.1 The advantages and disadvantages of reflecting alone or with others

Method of reflection	Possible advantages	Possible disadvantages
Alone	Easy to action – you can do it at any time as there is no need to arrange a meeting, etc. It can be lonely You have to be self-motivated to do it It can remain private and this may encourage honesty in the reflection	Your attention may wander New perspectives are less likely to emerge. Individuals often get stuck in a rut and habitually go over the same patterns of thought or visit the same dead ends The effectiveness of the reflection depends on your own level of self-awareness There is no opportunity for discussion, collaborative or shared learning
With a peer	The power differential between yourself and your peer is likely to be minimal and if it is a reciprocal arrangement this can help it to feel safe rather than exposed to 'judgement' A peer may be able to empathize with your situation most effectively It may be possible to reflect together on an experience that was shared by both parties People see things from different perspectives so this provides another perspective on the situation being discussed The fact that the process involves another person may be a motivation to reflect	The time and place may need to be prearranged and the logistics of this may be difficult If it is not reciprocal, it may feel exposing to share your reflections with someone else A peer who empathizes too closely with your situation may be reluctant to challenge your assumptions and preconceptions A peer may not have the experience or knowledge required to maximize learning from the reflective discussion
In a group of your peers	Provides plenty of alternative perspectives on the situation Can provoke learning through discussion and sharing	The logistics of getting a group of people together to reflect may be problematic A group setting may feel less safe

(Continued)

Table 5.1 continued

Method of reflection	Possible advantages	Possible disadvantages
With a facilitator	Provides another perspective on the situation being discussed The facilitator should be focused on helping you to reflect in a way that is most beneficial to your learning The facilitator may be in a position to facilitate you in taking your reflection forward, e.g. through appropriate reading or experience	There is likely to be a power imbalance between you and the facilitator and this may lead to lack of trust and defensiveness in the nature of the reflection The facilitator may not be available or willing to meet with you when it would be most useful to reflect
With your manager	The manager may be in a position to facilitate you in taking your reflection and learning forward, particularly through providing appropriate experience and environment	There is likely to be a power imbalance between yourself and the manager and this may lead to lack of trust and defensiveness in the nature of the reflection There may be some blurring of boundaries between the reflective discussions and formal appraisal mechanisms and this is unhelpful in encouraging the reflective process It may be difficult to get your manager to commit sufficient dedicated time to this activity Your manager may not fully understand the role for which you are being prepared and therefore may not be willing or able to facilitate your learning
Within Clinical Supervision	Your Clinical Supervisor should be trained to have the expertise to maximize your learning from the reflective discussion Regular Clinical Supervision provides time dedicated to your professional development and should provide continuity in the relationship with your supervisor	Not everyone has access to formal Clinical Supervision Your Clinical Supervisor may not fully understand the role for which you are being prepared and therefore may not be able to facilitate your learning Clinical Supervision sessions may be infrequent and may not be timed to occur when it would be most useful for you to reflect

Your role in facilitating reflection with others

Eliciting reflection or facilitating reflecting from another practitioner requires particular skills. It is amazing what can be learnt by helping others to reflect on their practice.

Some models of reflection are detailed enough to provide specific questions that colleagues can use to help each other deepen their reflection (Rolfe et al. 2001). However, beyond asking such questions there are a variety of ways in which reflective partners can operate, and below are suggestions of helpful roles that the 'other person' can play when reflecting in pairs (Allin and Turnock 2007).

- *Listener*: just listens – giving the 'reflector' the opportunity to think aloud.

- *Sounding board*: listens and responds to any questions the reflector may ask.

- *Summarizer:* repeats key phrases, summarizes, asks for clarification.

- *Buddy*: notices, empathizes, supports, and possibly advises.

- *Coach*: agrees objectives, provides feedback, and asks questions that assist reflection.

- *Interviewer (with a script)*: asks set questions or follows a certain review sequence.

- *Child*: just keeps asking 'why?' The reflector can stop the process at any point.

- *Devil's advocate*: tests and challenges what the reflector says. This needs careful briefing to ensure that the challenges are perceived as being part of a helpful process.

Choosing a medium for joint reflection

If you are going to reflect with others, then it is worth considering how this will be accomplished. In Chapter 1 we explored the role of formalized action learning in structuring group reflection and problem solving. Here we consider the practicalities of a range of different mediums. Often the logistics of arranging face-to-face meetings when location and full diaries are against you means that it may be preferable to use e-technology as a vehicle for discussions. These can take place on-line using written dialogue, online discussion boards or by telephone or Skype technology.

Each medium has advantages and disadvantages. Some lend themselves to sharing written reflections with others to promote discussion. Some may use a combination of both as written reflections may be shared and then become the subject of on-line discussion or phone conversations. Plack, Dunfee, Rindflesch and Driscoll (2008) recommend the use of virtual learning groups as a strategy for collaboratively solving problems using reflection via asynchronous discussion online. They recommend that for maximum benefit these are facilitated by mentors, but if this is not possible, then you may wish to consider setting up more informal online collaborative reflection groups within your own peer networks on your FD course or in the workplace.

Simon, a first year FD student, shares his experiences of using a discussion board to support his learning

When I was undertaking the induction to my Foundation Degree I discovered how learning technologies can support group discussion and decision-making and assist with the process of reflection. I used a discussion board with my fellow students to develop my skills of discussion and by sharing my queries with other students on the discussion board I was able to understand the requirements of my Foundation Degree. It was a little daunting to begin with as the technology was new and I was not sure how to get the most out of using it. However, the course tutors provided structured events in which students were encouraged to discuss key questions related to practice, wider reading, political issues impacting on our practice, and core learning for each module. In one module we were formatively assessed on a discussion board issue related to a learning outcome for that module. As we grew in confidence, it became an integral part of our own individual learning and that of the entire group. It enabled us to debate and critique key issues which helped us to engage with deeper forms of learning.

This chapter has introduced a range of tools which could aid your reflection and the choice of whether to reflect alone or with others. In Chapter 6, we will discuss how you can use learning contracts and action plans to evidence your learning in the workplace.

Key learning points

- Reflection is a skill for lifelong learning which enables learning from experience.

- Developing your skills as a reflective learner takes time and practice but is time well spent.

- Both reflection 'in action' and 'on action' are important and may both be evidenced in writing activities on your FD course.

- Critical incident analysis is a useful vehicle for reflection and any incident can potentially be a critical incident you can learn from.

- There are a variety of models of reflective practice that may be used to guide and structure your reflection. Try them out and choose what suits you best.

- A wide variety of experiences may provide a catalyst for your reflection. Seek them out and make use of them.

- Your creative and imaginative powers can be harnessed to stimulate reflection and learning.

- Reflexivity enhances learning from reflection, increases self-awareness and thereby improves practice.

- Reflection may take place alone or with others and in a variety of ways. They each have advantages and disadvantages so try as many forms as you can.

- You have a role to play in helping others to reflect. Hone the skills you need to do this and both you and your learning partner(s) will learn more.

- Take steps to maintain confidentiality and anonymity within any reflective writing.

Critical review questions
- **How can you use reflective writing to enhance your practice?**
- **Are your aware of your own values and beliefs and how these may impact on your practice?**
- **How could you promote reflective practice within your workplace?**

Reading for interest

Driscoll, J. (ed.) (2007) *Practising Clinical Supervision: A Reflective Approach for Healthcare Professionals*, 2nd edn. Edinburgh: Baillière Tindall.

References

Allin, L. and Turnock, C. (2007) *Reflection on and in the Workplace*. Reflection Students.

Driscoll, J. (ed.) (2007) *Practising Clinical Supervision: A Reflective Approach for Healthcare Professionals*, 2nd edn. Edinburgh: Baillière Tindall.

Ghaye, T. and Lillyman, S. (2006) *Learning Journals and Critical Incidents: Reflective Practice for Health Care Professionals*, 2nd edn. London: Quay Books.

Jasper, M. (2006) *Professional Development, Reflection, and Decision Making*. Oxford: Blackwell.

Plack, M.M., Dunfee, H., Rindflesch, A. and Driscoll, M. (2008) Virtual action learning sets: a model for facilitating reflection in the clinical setting. *Journal of Physical Therapy Education*, 22(3): 33–41.

Rolfe, G., Freshwater, D. and Jasper, M. (2001) *Critical Reflection for Nursing and the Helping Professions: A User's Guide*. Basingstoke: Palgrave.

Schön, D. (1991) *The Reflective Practitioner: How Professionals Think in Action*. Aldershot: Arena Ashgate Publishing Ltd.

Winter, R., Buck, A. and Sobiechowska, P. (1999) *Professional Experience and the Investigative Imagination*. London: Routledge.

6 How do you use learning contracts and action plans to demonstrate learning in the workplace?

Barbara Workman

Introduction

In Chapter 5 we demonstrated how you can use a range of different tools to help you to develop your skills in reflecting in and on practice. One of the fundamental methods used to help you evidence learning in the workplace is a learning contract. A learning contract will enable you to structure your learning activities as part of your FD course. However, they are also generally a useful tool to enable you to think about structuring your learning during your annual appraisal with your workplace manager.

Upon completion of this chapter, you should be able to do the following:

1 **Identify how a learning contract and an action plan can be used to enhance your learning in practice.**

2 **Plan your own learning contract and identify your role and that of your workplace mentor and course tutor in developing, implementing and evaluating your learning contract and/or action plans.**

3 **Outline key challenges to gaining support for completing your learning contract in practice and how these might be overcome.**

4 **Identify the ethical issues associated with developing a learning contract that focuses on the workplace and how these might be managed.**

When would you use a learning contract?

As part of your FD you may be required to develop a learning contract (LC) with your tutor and workplace mentor. This will enable you to identify clear learning goals which may be tied to your job description, skills, competencies and applying specific new course knowledge to your workplace. Some FD courses may require you to complete an LC as part of a theoretical assessment or it may form part of a reflective portfolio. An LC is designed to suit your own learning needs, but also needs to meet university, professional or employer requirements. Your FD course will determine the academic level required, and your employer or profession will determine the performance criteria. This means that LCs in the workplace may be a mixture of academic knowledge and practical skills. Your tutor will support both you and your mentor to design the appropriate learning objectives for your LC. It may take you some time to draft the contract until you feel you have agreed objectives that work for you. The benefits of LCs usually outweigh the challenges, as it will help you to 'learn how to learn' (Doncaster 2000), increase your motivation, build your confidence and ability to learn by yourself, and help you to link new knowledge to your workplace (Munroe et al. 2008).

If you refer to the learning contract example in Figure 6.1 you will notice that it has a structured layout.

Name: F. Tuck   **Programme: FD Health and Social Care, Rehabilitation**

Placement: Stroke Unit   Date: March–June

Learning Outcomes	Programme Learning outcome: Understanding and meeting nutritional needs. My Learning Outcome: Exploring and meeting nutritional needs of stroke clients
Resources	Placement protocols, dietician, speech therapist, visit by nutritional support rep, mentor, library, intranet – local policies
Learning activities	Care plans, supporting clients at mealtimes, observed visits/client assessments, supervised practice, observe nasogastric tube insertion and aftercare, percutaneous endoscopic gastrostomy insertion and aftercare, nutrition project
Assessment mode	Demonstrate competence in feeding support, portfolio completion, case study demonstrating appropriate nutrition, evidence-based intervention, demonstrate evidence of integration and application of new knowledge to practice
Evidence required	Portfolio: completed feeding support competency, competence statements, observed practice for feeding and supplements, case study and nutrition project, example care plans

First review date:

Mid-term review:

Final comments:

Learner's signature: Date:

Mentor/assessor signature: Date:

Tutor signature: Date:

Figure 6.1 Example of a learning contract

Figure 6.1 includes the following sections:

- Your name and programme: this is the unique identifier to ensure the correct course outcomes and expectations are used.

- Workplace location and dates: this ensures that the learning outcomes match the workplace opportunities, for type and length of experience.

- Learning outcomes: these may include programme learning outcomes for the workplace from which your specific learning needs are identified to reflect learning opportunities available at work.

- Resources: these include people and available resources, e.g. specialists, protocols.

- Learning activities: e.g. visits to the multi-disciplinary team, specialist client care, treatment activities.

- Assessment mode: this may be a mix of competencies and academic activities.

- Evidence required: e.g. records of practical skills, practice opportunities, care plans.

- Signatures of learner, mentor, and tutor.

A good LC has regular reviews built in to allow you to monitor your progress and make adjustments where required. The sample LC demonstrates the link between methods of assessment and the evidence of learning achieved. Linking personal, professional and workplace goals will ensure that your LC is robust.

To demonstrate this further it is important to understand the inter-relationship between yourself as learner, your mentor, your course tutor and your employer. Figure 6.2 outlines the roles and responsibilities of each in turn. You should all work together to ensure through the LC that a high standard of performance is evidenced for the assessment process.

As a learner, your responsibility is to actively seek out learning opportunities and resources. You will need to take the initiative to get feedback from your mentor and review your own progress against the agreed outcomes. This may appear a bit daunting at first but if you take the initiative to get feedback from your mentor, you

The learner	Identify own learning needs, agree learning activities, undertake learning, prepare for assessment, practise for competence, maintain portfolio
Mentor/assessor	Agree learning outcomes to meet learning needs, identify learning opportunities, provide, facilitate, and monitor learning activities in the workplace, assess learning and provide feedback
Tutor/university	Teach learner and mentor to use LCs, set standard of required academic performance, oversee and record assessment process and outcomes, provide learning support for learner and mentor
Employer/profession	Identify competence requirements, provide learning opportunities, provide trained mentors and assessors, agree skills required for job role

Figure 6.2 Roles and responsibilities of each person in the learning contract

can review your progress on a regular basis against the agreed learning outcomes. Your tutor and mentor will help to plan your LC and as you progress through your course it will get easier as you get more experienced and you may find that your LC begins to link with the previous one. Most assessments will be determined by the programme and competency requirements, but you may be able to negotiate the assignment topic so that it relates to your workplace.

Fatima, an FD graduate, shows how her organizational skills have benefitted from using a learning contract.

Time management was not one of my strong points when I started the Foundation Degree and I must admit I was rather worried about how I would juggle work, life and study. However, the use of a learning contract really helped me organize my learning in the workplace. It enabled me to clearly identify the skills I needed to develop and how I would achieve my goals. But, most importantly for me it has ensured that I prioritize my goals and set a realistic number that I can achieve within a designated timeframe. I used to be too ambitious and end up being disappointed because I could not achieve all I had set out to achieve. Using a learning contract on the FD course has helped me to develop my organizational skills and to become a better planner.

Another way of managing workplace learning is through the use of **action plans**.

When would you use an action plan?

Action plans are focused, setting goals with very specific activities so that it is clear when something has been achieved. They differ from LCs because they set priorities and include opportunities for personal reflection on progress. Figure 6.3 provides an example of a completed action plan. You will notice that it includes:

- skills to be acquired;
- actions to be taken;
- the resources needed;
- timeframe for completion;
- possible problems and reflections.

The action plan enables you to be clear that you have all the resources you need and a realistic timeframe to achieve the goals you have set for yourself. In order to achieve maximum success in using an action plan, we outline here some important tips which you may find helpful in developing a sample plan of your own. This is important because when you first set out to plan your learning, you are often over-ambitious and bite off more than you can chew. To effectively use an action plan to manage your learning you need to ensure that your goals are *s*pecific, *m*easurable, *a*chievable, *r*ealistic and *t*imed (SMART). SMART objectives are explored in more detail in Chapter 7 and we link this to Personal Development Planning. The following Time Out activity enables you to devise your own action plan.

Skills to be acquired	Providing oral care for client with dysphagia
Actions to take	Identify client to work with, practise oral care skills, read oral policy and discuss with mentor, ask mentor to assess my progress, book assessment
Resources needed	Mentor to identify appropriate client, oral skills demonstration and practice, oral policy documents
Timeframe	3–4 weeks
Possible problems/reflective comments	No suitable clients currently, discuss with mentor Have given oral care before – how much do I need to relearn?

Figure 6.3 Example of an action plan

Time Out: Devising your own action plan

Review the demands of your course, work or home life over the next few weeks. Devise an action plan to organize your priorities, anticipating some potential problems or opportunities that lie ahead.

Ask yourself these questions:

- *What* must be achieved?
- *How* will I do it? e.g. resources
- *When* must this be done by?
- *Who* can help me?
- *Where* does it happen?
- *How* important or urgent is it?
- *What* might distract me from my goals?

Use the action plan template provided below to help you answer these questions.

Skills to be acquired	
Actions to take	
Resources needed	
Timeframe	
Possible problems/ reflective comments	

The creation of a learning contract or an action plan depends very much on working effectively with a range of people to gain support for your learning in the workplace. We will now explore this in more detail.

How do you find effective support for work based learning?

There are many people you can call upon to support your learning in the workplace but the most frequently used sources are your workplace mentor, your colleagues, clients and fellow students. Here we explore how to make the most of gaining their support for your learning.

Working with a mentor

When you start your FD course, you may experience higher levels of stress and anxiety than usual. This may in turn make it difficult for you to take in and retain new information, however, some people adapt quicker to change than others. One way to support you during this time would be to work closely with your mentor. During the induction process to your FD course, you will have had the opportunity to identify your learning and development needs with your mentor and tutor as discussed in Chapter 3.

Your mentor is responsible for supporting and facilitating your learning experience. The following tips might help you make the most of learning opportunities available in your workplace:

- Your mentor may alert you to something in particular, e.g. a client's skin condition, if the client is distressed, or any change in mobility. Watch and think carefully about what you are observing: is this usual? Why might this be happening? How important is this? Why has my attention been drawn to it?

- Ask questions either during the activity if appropriate or afterwards.

- When planning your LC, discuss what you already know and what you need to learn. Think about this before you meet and have your programme outcomes to hand and some ideas of your own.

- Find out the frequency and expectations of progress meetings.

- Seek out and agree learning opportunities with your mentor, e.g. a visit to another department to follow a client may need permission and arranging with your mentor.

- Keep a list of questions to ask, so that you use discussion time effectively.

- Mentors have their own responsibilities to complete, so be sensitive to other demands on their time. Quietly observe their interactions with other people and situations. Ask questions later about why certain decisions were made.

- In a difficult situation, watch your mentor dealing with it, and offer to carry out errands to help. Discuss it later when things are calmer to learn from it.

How do you overcome challenges in your mentor relationship?

Very occasionally you may find it difficult to work with a specific mentor. This can usually be resolved by politely explaining to them what you find difficult. For example, if you find him or her impatient, you could check that you have not misunderstood instructions or done something inappropriate. It may be that they are not aware of the impression that they are giving, and a gentle explanation on how you are feeling might help. Use assertive techniques and explain how you feel, e.g. 'I wonder if I have misunderstood you, I'm not sure if I am doing this right.' This gives them the opportunity to consider how you have been working together, without feeling criticized. Sometimes personalities clash, and the workplace manager or link course tutor may need to help resolve differences. Such situations are rare, but will affect your learning as you may feel uncomfortable at work. It also takes courage, tact and assertive skills to raise such issues and these may not be easy for you. Sometimes it is easier to gravitate towards a mentor at work that you feel a natural rapport with. Learning to work with others is part of integrating into a profession, and developing self-awareness will help.

If you cannot resolve the issues you have with your mentor, and you can demonstrate evidence that you have indeed tried to find a solution, it is important that you work with your employer and tutor to find an alternative mentor. Some of the common reasons why people change their mentor include:

- Work roster clashes where there is minimal opportunity to work with your mentor.

- Mismatched expectations of what you will achieve on your course which cannot be resolved.

- A desire to work with an alternative mentor who has a different skill set.

- Maternity or sickness absence.

Try the following Time Out activity to help you think through how you may address potential issues in the mentor relationship.

Time Out: Addressing issues in your relationship with your mentor

Talking to other students on your FD course you discover that they are spending more time with their mentor than you and that their mentor is actively supporting their learning by providing a range of opportunities outside of the workplace. You realize that you need to address this situation to ensure that your learning is not affected. What actions would you consider?

You may have considered a range of actions but remember that there are people who can help you resolve the situation.

Fatima, a FD graduate, shares her experiences of how she resolved her conflict with a workplace mentor during her course.

At the beginning of my course I found my workplace mentor very difficult to work with. We found that we had very different approaches to what was required of the FD course, different styles and ways of working and experienced issues with trying to work on the same shift pattern. There were quite a few workplace issues that were happening at the time which made an increasing demand on her time and attention so I sat down with her and my manager and the course tutor, to explore the issues. This helped me to identify and reiterate my expectations of the relationship, and my manager and course tutor supported me to arrange another workplace mentor who had more time to devote to my development during the course. The matter was resolved swiftly, amicably and positively for all concerned as my first mentor was very anxious about letting me down. The important learning point I would like to share with all FD students is to ensure that you resolve problems swiftly and early on in your development, don't leave things to fester and build up as they become more difficult to resolve and impact negatively on your own learning.

Working with clients, colleagues and fellow students

Everyone has been a learner in a new situation and most people are keen to share their knowledge and experience. If you are unsure about what to do, ask for help rather than hoping that you will just find out. Some of the most useful learning will come from your clients, or their families. When working with clients, ask their viewpoints and experience. If they have a chronic condition, they will be experts on managing their daily living activities. If it is an acute condition, ask how they are coping, what their concerns are, what sort of things they liked doing when well and at home. These conversations can give you insights into what it is like being cared for, and can inform your future practice and understanding. It can also give you clues about motivating clients during their recovery.

Your FD course may have assignments that allow you to explore client case studies in detail, so gaining an understanding of the lived experience of clients and their families is an important part of your learning in and from the workplace. Discussions with colleagues and fellow students are good learning opportunities too. Recounting events from work can help make sense of the situation, and other people's explanations and stories give you additional knowledge. Reflecting on incidents and discussing them with friends and family can help your understanding. Be careful though as to where these conversations take place. If held in a public place, private information may be heard by a casual listener which may be inappropriate. You should consider confidentiality of information about others, wherever you share it. That includes talking with colleagues while caring for a client. Make sure you include the client in the conversation, even if they are not able to join in. They do not want to know the intimate details of your night out, or of another client's treatment!

Simon demonstrates how he has been able to develop his workplace practice as a result of working with others.

Before I commenced the Foundation Degree I did not have the confidence to share my experiences with other colleagues. I felt that as a Health Care Assistant I had little knowledge to share in discussions with registered professionals within the team. My attitude began to change as I developed more confidence in my understanding and application of the theory which underpinned the care I deliver to my client group in the workplace. Gradually, with encouragement from my mentor and course tutors, I have begun to share my observations with colleagues in the workplace through handover reports, case conferences and journal clubs, and with my peers through my action learning group. It has given me the confidence to share my observations, to question my own practice and to ensure that the care I give is based on the best available evidence.

What are the ethical issues associated with work based learning?

As discussed in Chapter 5, all evidence of learning from the workplace should consider ethical issues of confidentiality so that colleagues' and clients' identities are not revealed without their express permission. If anyone contributes information for your evidence or projects, tell them how you will use the information and who will have access to it. Data from clients or notes should only be used for the purpose for which it was collected, and is covered by the Data Protection Act (1998), so should not breach the rights of others and must be anonymous. Information and ideas that belong to other people, and which may result from work activities, are their **intellectual property** or that of your organization, and therefore you should ask permission to use them as part of your evidence. Permission may be required for other sorts of evidence too, so check with your tutor before including it.

This chapter has introduced you to learning contracts and action plans and who can support your learning in the workplace. In Chapter 7 we will discuss the use of personal development plans to demonstrate your development in the workplace.

Key learning points

- Learning contracts will enable you to identify clear learning outcomes which are linked to your job description, skills competencies and underpinning knowledge.

- A good learning contract includes regular review meetings and demonstrates a link between methods of assessment and learning achieved.

- For an action plan to be effective, you need to make sure that the goals are specific, measurable, achievable, realistic and timed (SMART).

- Remember that working with a mentor will allow you to link theory and practice. However, not all relationships work and there are other people who can support you in addressing these issues.

- Clients, their families and colleagues provide a range of learning opportunities but confidentiality must be maintained at all times.

Critical review questions
- How would you incorporate a learning contract in the workplace?
- What role could an action plan have in facilitating your WBL?
- How could you use clients and their families to support your learning at and for work?

Web links and useful resources

Higher Education Academy.
http://www.engsc.ac.uk/er/theory/learning.asp

Reading for interest

Anderson, G., Boud, D. and Sampson, J. (1996) *Learning Contracts: A Practical Guide*. London: Kogan Page.
Wilson, S. and Dobson, M. (2008) *Goal Setting: How to Create an Action Plan and Achieve Your Goals*, 2nd edn. New York: American Management Association.

References

Doncaster, K. (2000) Learning agreements: their function in work-based programmes at Middlesex University. *Education and Training*, 42(6): 349–55, available at: http://www.emerald-library.com.
Kolb, D. (1984) *Experiential Learning*. New York: Prentice Hall.
Munroe, M., Holmshaw, J. and Brown, V. (2008) *Review of literature on the impact of learning contracts on teaching and learning in higher education institutions*. Unpublished report, Centre for Excellence in Work Based Learning, Middlesex University.

7 | How do you use Personal Development Plans to demonstrate learning in the workplace?

Claire Thurgate

Introduction

This chapter will help you to develop an effective Personal Development Plan (PDP) to demonstrate your learning in the workplace. It helps you to develop the skills of organizing, structuring, writing and evaluating your PDP using a range of hints and tips. It explains how you can use your PDP to demonstrate your development during annual appraisal, as well as identifying how you can structure it to include **National Occupational Standards** (NOS) and competencies. The chapter also explores the importance of the relationship with your **mentor**, employer and course tutors who play an important role in helping you to develop your PDP.

Upon completion of this chapter, you should be able to do the following:

1 Identify the key elements of a PDP.

2 Write your own PDP as part of your FD course.

3 Implement your PDP in the workplace.

4 Evaluate the impact of your PDP on your own learning.

Why do you need to develop a PDP?

If you work in the health and social care sector there is an expectation that you will progress your career and develop your self continually throughout your professional working life in order to ensure that you are fit for purpose. Your PDP will enable you to demonstrate to your employer the range of **transferable skills** you have developed. Transferable skills, also known as *graduate* or *key skills*, include team work, oral or written communication skills, problem solving, and critical thinking skills. They are generic core skills that you have developed that can be transferred to any other work context to help you undertake your role.

A PDP is a useful tool to enable you to reflect the changing context of your work as well as your changing knowledge and skill base. Your PDP will help you identify your personal development goals and evaluate your progress in achieving these. A PDP is designed to provide a baseline for ongoing personal development and therefore life-long learning. It is often referred to as cyclical because you plan, implement and evaluate your goals and whether you have achieved them. This process is outlined in Figure 7.1. You will notice from Figure 7.1 that it shares a similar structure to the learning contracts that we discussed in Chapter 6 (Figure 6.1). It requires you to identify an area of development, the action and resources you need to meet your development, an account of what evidence you will use to demonstrate achievement and an evaluation and reflection based on your achievements so that you may identify further development needs.

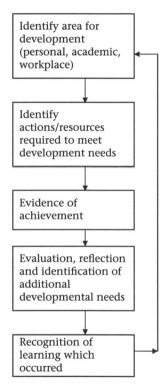

Figure 7.1 The cyclical process involved in PDP
Source: QAA (2009).

You should aim to be aware of areas within your personal and professional life that require development. For example, you may have difficulty remembering how to reference appropriately for a course assignment, or you may need to develop the skill of undertaking a new procedure within the workplace. If these areas of improvement are not formally captured within a PDP, then they will be forgotten. As a result, you will be unable to evaluate whether you have improved your practice or knowledge base and demonstrate what was learnt during the process. Therefore, a PDP allows you to capture areas for development formally, and evaluate and summarize what learning has been achieved.

A PDP may also be used to provide relevant evidence to support career development and demonstrate competency within the workplace. The process of identifying areas which you wish to develop will be similar to those discussed above. The difference may be related to the time that it takes to collect the appropriate evidence and the different forms of evidence required. If, for example, you identified that your goal is to become a Band 4 Assistant Practitioner (AP), then it is likely that the evidence needed will be the successful completion of a course of academic study, such as a two-year Foundation Degree. Or it may be that you need to demonstrate competence in a particular AP role. Therefore, you are likely to use both long- and short-term goals. Sub-dividing a long-term goal into shorter more manageable objectives will enable you to evaluate your achievements on a regular basis and may allow you to tackle something which looks rather ambitious in smaller chunks of activity which are achievable. This will allow you to gain a sense of achievement and motivation to achieve the bigger, longer-term goals.

What does a PDP look like?

A PDP is likely to be initiated following an appraisal, a change in your role or because you are undertaking a course of study. If you work in the NHS, the appraisal review process formally identifies areas for development which are linked to the **Knowledge and Skills Framework** (KSF) (DH 2004). Figures 7.2 and 7.3 provide you with an example of a FD student's PDP for enhancing her communication skills with the multi-disciplinary team. It shows how she intends to develop her Band 4 AP role through attendance at team meetings, appraisal, her FD course or the learning that she undertakes on her FD course and through interaction with her peers, work colleagues and client group.

As your PDP is linked to your appraisal, role development or course of study, it is a more formal way of monitoring and evidencing your development and as a result it may consist of a number of components, including action plans, learning contracts or excerpts from your reflective diary. This evidence, like your PDP, is personal to you. Your course, employer or workplace may require you to develop a portfolio of learning of which your PDP will be a component part. Depending on local practice, your portfolio may be in a paper or electronic format.

Relevant dimensions	**Communication** Communicate with a range of people on a range of matters.
What is the development need/interest?	Now that I have a Band 4 Associate Practitioner role I am required to communicate with the multi-disciplinary team
What will I do to develop myself?	I will take responsibility for communicating changes to the multi-disciplinary team. I will contribute to team meetings.
How will I know I have done this?	I will have discussed changes with the multi-disciplinary team. I feel confident talking during team meetings.
What is the date for planned completion?	Six months
What support do I need and where will I get it?	I need support to increase my self-confidence to talk to members of the multi-disciplinary team. I will work with my manager who does my appraisal. I hope that my confidence will improve as a result of the knowledge which I will gain doing my Foundation Degree.
What are the barriers and how can I overcome them?	Not always working with my manager. I need to find someone else to work with on the days I do not work with my manager. I am shy. I will talk to student study support at the university as communication is a graduate skill which I need to develop as part of my Foundation Degree.

Figure 7.2 PDP template to meet the NHS KSF
Source: DoH (2004).

Relevant dimensions	Communication Communicate with a range of people on a range of matters.
Learning and development activity	To lead a discussion on a patient's condition with the nurse in charge and the Occupational Therapist.
Hours and dates	1000-1100, 18 December 2011
Has the learning activity been (a) completed? (b) effective ?	The learning activity was completed effectively.
How will you apply this learning to your work?	When I am discussing a patient with others I will make sure that I am fully aware of the patient's condition and any changes. I will make sure that I ask questions to help me understand any changes to a patient's care.
Who else could you share this learning with?	I will share this learning with - other Associate Practitioners - colleagues who are undertaking the Foundation Degree with me as not all of them work in the health sector - senior healthcare assistants - newly qualified professionals - new staff to the ward who may not be used to leading team discussions

Figure 7.3 PDP record and evaluation to meet the NHS KSF
Source: DoH (2004).

The following Time Out activity allows you to reflect on your achievements in the last year in preparation for your appraisal and writing a PDP:

Time Out: Preparing for annual appraisal

Prior to your annual appraisal you need to complete any preparatory paperwork which may include such questions as:

- **Looking back, what have you achieved in the last year? The examples you give may be general if you have not had a formal appraisal before. Or, if you have had a formal appraisal, then your examples need to link to some identified learning objectives.**
- **Looking forwards, what do you want to achieve in the next year? This is where you might link your development goals to your job description, a KSF if you are working within the health sector and any National Occupational Standard. You will need to consider what evidence you will provide to demonstrate achievement.**

Once you have completed the Time Out activity, you will have a good starting point for a PDP. You may review this throughout the year or at your mid-way appraisal and as a result of this review process you will adapt, amend and complete aspects of your PDP. From these achievements you will identify additional learning goals which you need to achieve and hence you will be engaging with the cyclical process of PDP as outlined in Figure 7.1.

Fatima, an FD graduate student, describes how she engaged with PDP since completing her course.

During my annual appraisal my manager would set goals which I needed to achieve over the year. However, I must admit, when I look back, I did not always have a clear plan regarding how I would achieve these goals or why I needed to undertake this specific development. These attitudes have now changed as a result of the Foundation Degree and I understand the need to engage in personal development and Life Long Learning. The use of a structured PDP has really helped me to focus on specific goals, provide appropriate evidence and ultimately enhance the care which I provide. I use the evidence that I collect during the year to discuss with my manager to show her what I have achieved during my appraisal and catch up meetings.

If you are undertaking a course currently your PDP will need to demonstrate a number of key criteria which are pre-determined by the **Quality Assurance Agency** (2009). Your PDP must be:

- *Discrete* – your PDP is personal to you and should be designed according to your specific learning needs with support from your course tutors.

- *Linked* – your PDP may have specific links to the modules which you are studying, for example, your course may cover PDP in academic skills sessions or require you to complete a personal reflective diary or a learning contract which is linked to your PDP.

- *Embedded* – PDP is a specific requirement of your course and is embedded in the course learning outcomes.

- *Integrated* – learning activities throughout your course are linked to the development of your PDP and learning within your workplace. Therefore, course tutors and mentors have a responsibility for supporting your PDP.

- *Extended* – your PDP will enable you to integrate broader learning activities which have occurred outside of your course or workplace, for example, voluntary work or hobbies.

How do you write a PDP?

A useful starting point for your PDP is to undertake a SWOT (Strengths, Weaknesses, Opportunities and Threats) analysis. This will help you to undertake a detailed review of your skills and strengths and where you are in your career currently. You can work through it on your own or with the help of your mentor or a group of colleagues. The aim is to help you note down as many of the strengths, weaknesses/challenges, opportunities and threats associated with your current role as you can. How you approach this will vary depending on the type of learner you are, which you will have identified in Chapter 3. The list below identifies some of the criteria you may use to guide your analysis:

* *Strengths and weakness of your role* – relate to your knowledge, skills, experience, expertise, decision-making, communication skills, interprofessional relationships, time-keeping, organizational or practical skills.

* *Opportunities* – your experience in previous employment or potential strengths you feel you may have.

* *Threats* – may include factors and circumstances that prevent you from achieving your goals for personal, professional or career development, or service improvements.

Figure 7.4 shows you a commonly used tool to help you keep notes for your analysis.

Undertake the following Time Out activity to enable you to apply the principles of SWOT analysis to your own development.

Strengths	Weaknesses
Opportunities	Threats

Figure 7.4 SWOT analysis

Time Out: Identifying learning objectives from your SWOT analysis

* **Using the SWOT box in Figure 7.4, note down strengths, weaknesses, opportunities and threats in your current role.**
* **From this analysis identify three learning objectives to enhance your role development. These might be related objectives for your FD course or areas you wish to discuss at your appraisal.**

Specific goal	Writing
Measurable	Hand in first assignment
Achievable	I need to write the assignment to pass the module
Realistic	I can use the computer to help me get my assignment written in time
Time-bound	Must be submitted at the end of my first term

Figure 7.5 Alice's first PDP for her academic skills module

Once you have completed your SWOT analysis, you are ready to write your PDP. When writing learning goals for your PDP, it is important that they follow SMART principles. This means that your objective must be Specific, Measurable, Achievable, Realistic and Time bound. The following Time Out activity presents a student's PDP as part of her FD course and will help you to write your own PDP. This is linked to the PDP in Figures 7.5 and 7.6.

Specific goal	To write in the third person
Measurable	First assignment will be written in the third person
Achievable	With the support of student study support and my tutor I will be able to write in the third person
Realistic	Writing in the third person is a requirement of my university course so I will need to begin as I am mean to go on.
Time-bound	I will complete my first assignment in the third person for the submission date
Evidence of achievement	Assignment was completed in the third person
Learning	I am usually very stubborn in relation to asking for help. However, accessing student study support made me realize that by asking for help in the beginning and addressing my concerns would save me time in the long term.

Figure 7.6 Alice's amended PDP for her academic skills module following discussions with her module leader

Time Out: Writing your PDP

Alice is undertaking her first module on a FD course where she has been asked to develop a PDP as part of her assessment. As Alice is concerned about her writing skills, she decides to focus on this for her PDP. She undertakes a SWOT analysis where she identifies her strengths and weaknesses with her writing, the opportunities that the course might present her with to improve her writing skills, and the negative experiences she has had in writing academic assignments in the past. From the SWOT analysis she develops her

PDP to discuss with her tutor (see Figures 7.5 and 7.6). Figure 7.5 shows Alice's first attempt to develop a PDP. You can see that it is rather simplistic and does not use SMART principles effectively. Figure 7.6 shows what her PDP looks like once she has had a meeting with her course tutor. You can see that the learning objective is much more focused and specific. The measurement is altered to demonstrate that success will be achieved through writing academically against predetermined module criteria for assignments.

Thinking about your own development, identify one learning objective attached to your course or workplace needs and write your own PDP using SMART principles. Once you have completed this discuss it with your course tutor or mentor to get feedback.

The above Time Out activity demonstrates what a completed PDP may look like but what is important when you prepare your PDP is to develop the ability to ask yourself questions. Completing the following Time Out activity will help you consider what questions you should ask when you are developing your PDP.

Time Out: Preparing to write your PDP

Communication skills

The ability to communicate effectively and efficiently is vital when working in the health and social care sector. Therefore, consider:

- If you are able to communicate appropriately with different groups of people i.e. those with learning disabilities or are sight impaired.
- How people interpret your body language. Is your list similar to a colleagues list regarding your body language?

Working with others

Working in health and social care involves working with a number of other professionals. To work effectively you need to consider:

- Are you able to listen to others' needs and change your ways of working as a result?
- Do you take an active role when working with others?
- Are you able to overcome difficulties when working with others?
- Are you able to give feedback to colleagues or those from different teams?

Academic development

The aim of this component is to help you learn how to be an effective learner.

Academic skills

The university/college where you are studying may have an academic assessment test which you could complete to identify your strengths and weaknesses. You may also like to consider:

- Are you aware of the requirements for submitting an academic piece of work i.e. essay, report, PowerPoint presentation?
- Are you aware of what referencing format to use? Can you implement the required format?
- Are you able to access information from a range of sources and evaluate its reliability and credibility?
- Are you able to incorporate discussion, critical discussion and evidence of reading into your work?

Managing your own learning

To make the most of your academic skills, you need to manage your learning effectively. Therefore, consider:

- How you will organize your studies, work and leisure to deal with priorities and meet deadlines?
- What range of resources can you access to support your development? For example, student study support, workplace, personal tutor, further education college.

Workplace development

Whether you are undertaking a programme of study which recognizes your learning in the workplace or you are developing skills to promote career progression it is important to consider:

- What skills are outlined in your current job description? Are you able to demonstrate that you are competent in these skills?
- What skills could you develop to enhance your role?
- What skills do you need to develop to promote career progression? For example, this may be to prepare for a new job or to progress through a gateway in the KSF.

Following from the above Time Out activities and before you start writing your PDP you may have the following questions.

How many goals should I include?

The number of goals required will vary depending upon why you are writing a PDP. If you need to use your PDP to evidence development in the workplace following your appraisal, then you may require three to five goals. As the appraisal cycle lasts a year, you could include long-term goals and short-term goals. If, however, you are using your PDP as part of a course of study and a module assessment, then one to three goals may be more realistic. Depending on the nature of the module and what progress you want to evidence, it is likely that you will have chosen short-term goals. For example, during your appraisal, you may have identified in your PDP that you want to become a Band 4 Assistant Practitioner and complete a FD. These are long-term goals. How you achieve these goals would then be evidence within shorter-term goals as part of your course PDP. For example, you may use your goals to identify specific knowledge and skills which are related to the module you are studying and your long-term goal of being a Band 4 Assistant Practitioner.

How do I write the goals?

As discussed earlier in the chapter, your PDP is personal to you and you will be writing goals that will allow you to meet your own personal targets and the best way for you to achieve this. It is important that you note where you are starting from so that you can measure your progress and note whether you are building on existing strengths or building new knowledge and skills. This was discussed earlier in the chapter regarding SMART principles. Therefore, to help you evaluate your achievements you will need to ensure that your goals are *specific* i.e. 'I will learn how to reference my first assignment correctly' rather than 'I will learn referencing'. This means that feedback from your first assignment will allow you to *measure* your achievement. This is an *achievable* goal as you will receive lectures on referencing and there will be additional information on the Virtual Learning Environment or via study support. This is a *realistic* goal as it is part of the content on your course and a requirement of the assessment. This goal will also be achieved within an appropriate *timeframe*. This goal could be written as: I will apply the Harvard referencing system to my first assignment on my FD course and evaluate my skill on feedback from the course tutor in December 2010.

Who writes the goals?

As your PDP is personal to you and owned by you, it is your responsibility to write the goals, how you aim to achieve these goals and the evidence required to demonstrate achievement. However, you are not alone and it is highly advisable to discuss your PDP goals with your mentor and/or course tutor. They will be able to guide you in developing your thoughts and may provide alternative suggestions in relation to the focus of your goal, outcomes, evidence and evaluation.

How long is a PDP?

As your PDP is cyclical, ongoing and personal to you, there is no prescribed length. As your goals are specific, it is likely that you will use an A4 piece of paper, or electronically if you are required to use an electronic tool. The number of plans that you develop will depend on why you are developing a PDP. If your PDP is a requirement of your annual appraisal, then it is likely that it may consist of one or two sides of A4. If, however, your PDP is a component of a course of study, then it is likely that you will have a new goals for each module you complete which identifies academic and role knowledge and skills development. It is the evidencing of achievement which will form the majority of your portfolio.

What evidence should you collect to demonstrate achievement of your personal development goals?

When you are designing your PDP and selecting your learning goals, it is important that you spend a bit of time ensuring that you can produce the appropriate evidence to demonstrate that learning has been achieved. The evidence you use could come from a range of sources, i.e. the workplace, from your programme of study or from your personal life. What is important is that you are able to discuss how the evidence allows you to demonstrate your development and what you have learnt. You can always discuss what evidence may be appropriate with your mentor or your course tutor. Here we outline some ideas for sources of evidence you may wish to include:

1 A reflective diary entry which demonstrates how you have dealt with a difficult situation which has had a positive outcome.

2 A survey from your workplace which demonstrates how your colleagues perceive your strengths.

3 Evidence of communication from a patient, client or their relatives which thanks you for the care you have given.

4 A reflection account which demonstrates an episode of group working which went well or one that did not go quite as expected.

5 A statement from a colleague which may outline your role in ensuring effective team working, for example, as a leader.

6 A copy of a poster or PowerPoint presentation that you have delivered as part of your FD course.

7 Your course grades and completed assignments.

8 A timetable of how you will meet the demands of studying, work and leisure.

9 Your job description.

10 An action plan outlining what competences you need to achieve.

11 Your KSF PDP paperwork if you work in the health sector.

12 Completed and signed competences which are appropriate to your role.

13 A reflection outlining how you achieved your competences.

You may also include:

- an action plan outlining which skills you would like to develop to enhance your role;

- a statement from a colleague which outlines how you have developed within the workplace;

- your CV.

As we stated earlier, these are examples of evidence that may also form an integral part of your professional portfolio. You are not required to share all the sources of evidence that you use to support your learning and reflection in and on practice, for example, you are not required to share the full contents of your reflective diary with your course tutor, mentor or colleagues. You can be selective about what sources provide the best available evidence to demonstrate achievement of your learning objectives.

Simon, a first year FD student, shares his experience of providing evidence for his PDP.

The first assignment on the Foundation Degree involved a reflective diary to demonstrate our learning. As this was the first time that I had undertaken this form of assessment, I included all of the excerpts. When I received my feedback, my tutor explained that in future reflective assignments there may be aspects of my writing which I did not want to share with my tutor or mentor. At first I disagreed as I was happy to share my thoughts, however, as I have progressed on the Foundation Degree I have realized that I did not actually wish to share everything I had written. For example, when I was reflecting on team working within my workplace, I understood that I did not want to share my observations of the ward manager with my mentor. I had observed that my manager did not provide encouraging feedback to the team when we had worked hard and that this affected morale within the team. I felt that if I shared this with my mentor, that she would report this to my manager and I could get into trouble

How do you evaluate your PDP with your mentor/course tutor?

The final stage of the PDP cycle is to evaluate your achievements. This action is required for a number of reasons:

- to ensure that goals set are achieved;

- to identify what has been learnt including formal and informal learning;

- to identify areas for improvement;

- to consider whether any changes are required (i.e. was the plan realistic?);

- to outline future development needs.

An important part of designing a PDP in its earliest form is giving consideration to how you evaluate whether learning has taken place. Although it might seem out of order, an effective evaluation needs to be considered at the start of setting any objectives. This will allow you to identify appropriate evidence to demonstrate learning. Therefore, we recommend that when you are developing your initial goals for your PDP, you should discuss evaluation with the person who will be supporting you in this process. This may be your mentor or course tutor or both. During the initial discussion you should consider:

- how frequently you meet;

- how the meetings will be documented;

- whether you need to identify an associate mentor to work with if your main mentor is not available;

- how you will demonstrate and evaluate your development both in written format as part of a course assignment and when you attend meetings with your mentor and course tutor.

As discussed earlier in the chapter, your PDP can be linked to your appraisal and help with career planning, professional development and future career aspirations. You should be able to use it as evidence for your annual appraisal or to demonstrate that you have met the NOS requirements or evidence as career enhancement mapped against the KSF. In other words, PDP should become an integral part of your LLL and not just part of a course. Figure 7.7 provides an example of how PDP can be linked to annual appraisal. The following case study sets the context for Harry's PDP.

Case Study: Linking PDP to appraisal and career planning

Harry has worked with people who are visually impaired for five years and is aware of the publication *Good Practice Sight Guide* (RNIB 2008). He wants his work to reflect the areas of service delivery covered in the guide and therefore discusses this at his appraisal. His manager states that Harry's idea to meet the requirements of the *Good Practice Sight Guide* meet the needs of the organization and would be an appropriate focus for his PDP as it would enable him to demonstrate professional development within the organization. At the same time, the evidence which Harry collects would enable him to develop a portfolio which could be shared at an interview should Harry decide to progress his career and undertake a new role. Figure 7.7 demonstrates Harry's PDP following his appraisal.

Specific goal	To provide appropriate information to visually impaired service users, enabling them to make informed choices. (Good practice Benchmark 3)
Measurable	Information is provided in the service users' preferred format.
Achievable	By working with colleagues within my workplace and those from other disciplines I will be able to provide appropriate information in a format which is preferred by service users.
Realistic	This seems like a large task to achieve but I feel that if I split this into smaller goals that are continually evaluated, I will be able to achieve my outcome.
Time-bound	I have a year to achieve my goal. What I will do is break this into smaller time-bound goals which will ensure that I meet my outcome in the time scale given.

Figure 7.7 Harry's PDP following his appraisal

Harry's PDP (Figure 7.7) demonstrates how you can link your PDP to your professional development. It shows how the format Alice used (Figures 7.5 and 7.6) is versatile, irrespective of the focus or need of your PDP. However, when developing your PDP to demonstrate career progression or professional development, you may find that that you can divide your end goal into a number of smaller goals. This is an appropriate approach as it will allow you to evaluate your progress in achieving your goal and ensure that you obtain adequate evidence.

This chapter has introduced you to how you can use a PDP to demonstrate your development and how this may link to your LLL and career advancement. In Chapter 8, we will discuss why employers engage with work based learning as a way of developing their organization and quality of the service they provide.

Key learning points

- Your PDP is personal to you and will allow you to evidence achievement of knowledge and skills in the workplace or as part of a course of study. As a result, the content will vary from person to person.

- You need to identify specific developmental goals; actions; and sources to meet these; evidence of achievement and reflection on the process.

- Undertaking a SWOT analysis during the development phase of your PDP will allow you to identify where you are and where you want to be in terms of achieving your goals.

- Your PDP goals need to use SMART objectives.

- Long-term goals may be sub-divided into shorter-term goals.

> **Critical review questions**
> - How could the use of a PDP support your career development?
> - How do you write an effective PDP?
> - Who could support you in the development and achievement of your PDP?

Web links and resources

Providing health and social care policy, guidance and publications for NHS and social care professionals.
https://www.dh.gov.uk

Employer-led authority on the training standards and development needs for the social care sector.
https://www.skillsforcare.org.uk

Sector Skills Council for the UK health sector.
https://www.skillsforhealth.org.uk

Reading for interest

Cottrell, S. (2003) *Skills for Success: The Personal Development Planning Handbook*. Basingstoke: Palgrave Macmillan.

References

Department of Health (DoH) (2004) *The National Health Service Knowledge and Skills Framework (NHS KSF) and the Development Review Process*. London: Department of Health.
Quality Assurance Agency (QAA) (2009) *Personal Development Planning: Guidance for Institutional Policy and Practice in Higher Education*. London: Quality Assurance Agency.
Royal National Institute Blind (2008) 'Good Practice in Sight' Guide. London: RNIB'.

The benefits and challenges of learning in the workplace and future career development planning

8 | What are the benefits and challenges of work based learning for your employer?

Peter Ellis, Jane Abbott and Helen O'Keefe

Introduction

This chapter explores the benefits and challenges of work based learning (WBL) for your employing organization, and what your employer hopes you will gain from participating in a WBL programme such as a Foundation Degree. To understand why your learning matters to your organization, you need to understand how your organization sees you and the role that you play within it.

Upon completion of this chapter, you should be able to do the following:

1 Understand the potential benefits of WBL for your employer.

2 Identify the barriers to work based learning in the workplace and how these might be overcome.

3 Understand how to maximize support from your workplace managers and colleagues when planning to undertake WBL.

4 Demonstrate insight into the challenges of studying at Foundation Degree level.

What are the potential benefits of WBL for your employer?

WBL can help to improve partnership working and workplace support for learning and development which in turn reduces the cost of resources such as time, improves staff retention and the quality of care provided by the service. Each of these will be discussed in turn.

Partnership working for organizational learning

Organizations exist to get a job done. The size of organizations and the jobs that they do vary, but all organizations exist in order to further their own purposes (Seden 2003). In the health and social care sector, people are the purpose of the organization. The sort of work that is undertaken is often personal and the proximity to the people you care for is unlike that in any other professional group. Methods and approaches to care provision are constantly changing while the need for care is forever growing. Taking people away from the workplace for training and development puts an additional burden on services. WBL addresses the need for workers to be at work while learning, it allows the delivery of care to continue relatively uninterrupted, while allowing you to learn and develop to improve the quality of the care you provide.

Some organizations have cultures which actively promote learning and development and which recognize that investment in the education of their staff not only benefits them, but also their clients. These are known as **learning organizations**. Learning organizations are sustainable and flourish despite change and development, and it therefore makes sense for employers to adopt such a **learning culture** within their organization. Workplace culture and its impact upon your learning were explored in Chapter 2.

Investing in WBL means that your organization can develop at a pace and in a way that suits its needs. Embedding learning in the **organizational culture** means that education not only fits the **operational** needs of the organization, it can be adapted to fit its long-term developmental needs also. This is an important aspect of WBL because the proximity to the workplace means that the level, nature and content of the training can be aligned with the vision of the organization. This approach may be apparent within your FD course where you may have tasks identified by your employer which allow you to link the theory that you have learnt on your course to your role in the workplace. Some employers may link the development of your role competence to your job description. This ensures that your learning is very specific to the needs of your organization.

A good Foundation Degree will support a **tripartite** relationship between you, your employer and the higher education establishment which allows clear identification of individual roles. This approach ensures that the assessment of **competency** reflects the needs of the organization, while allowing you to achieve valid and transferable academic recognition for your achievements.

Saving time, money and promoting workplace support

By its very nature, WBL is also potentially financially cost effective for your organization. You are usually on site learning and working, you are not being paid to take time out to train, but can fit your training around the needs of your organization. Mentors are often drawn from within the existing workforce, perhaps people that have been through the same education and training as yourself or a recognized programme, i.e. nurse mentors, people who know and understand the work, but who also do not need to leave the workplace for long periods of time in order to facilitate training. The training and supervision of colleagues are of benefit to your manager and mentor, whose own learning and understanding are underpinned by the process of taking responsibility for the learning of others (Clouder 2009). Because of the inclusive nature of WBL, tools such as action plans, learning contracts and PDPs help you to situate your learning and gain support from your workplace mentor and course tutors. As it is tailored to the needs of your organization, and because of the involvement of management and supervision by your peers, there are real opportunities for your colleagues to be involved at different levels and in different ways in your development. Not only does this inclusivity benefit you as a student, but it helps to develop the skills of assessment and support among your mentors and also in team building, bonding and cohesion.

> **Cumulative knowledge: benefits of WBL versus other forms of training**
>
> - **Provides development opportunities for staff which is tailored to organizational need.**
> - **Generally cheaper than more conventional forms of training.**
> - **May be used to enable the team to learn together and therefore develop the team.**
> - **Less disruptive to the organization as students spend the majority of their time actually at work.**

Reduced staff turnover

WBL can help to improve staff recruitment and retention and general staff satisfaction. Motivational theorists have long understood that many workers are motivated by opportunities for training and development as much as they are by increased salary and promotion (Herzberg 1968). The philosophy of the Magnet Hospital project in the USA, Canada and Australasia, for example, demonstrates that staff who share the core values of their organization are more passionate about their work because they have a sense of belonging, and feel valued and empowered to take responsibility for the quality of service they provide. Worldwide research on workforce development shows that organizations that place learning and development at the heart of their endeavour have the highest quality of staff, provide the best quality of care, and are most able to adapt to changing health and social care contexts than those organizations that do not. The following Time Out activity will help you consider why WBL is beneficial to your organization.

> **Time Out: Benefits of WBL for an organization**
>
> At this stage, you might like to make a list of reasons as to why your employer should pay for you to engage in a course of WBL such as a Foundation Degree. Don't forget to list the benefits to the organization that you work for.

Making improvements in the quality of care

The Higher Education Academy (2006: 18) takes the view that there needs to be a re-emphasis 'on the need to "learn from real work"'. Caring work has many faces and requires the acquisition of many skills. Some of these skills come from the adoption of what Geertz (1973) calls **'common sense knowledge'**, that is, knowledge gained through, and in, practice. Certainly the ability to care will almost certainly develop in tandem with reflection on experience, but this reflection, or acquisition of common sense knowledge, needs a guiding hand. WBL enables you to acquire and build upon the knowledge you gain through experience by applying good educational practices to the process of learning through experience. For example, guided reflection and reading, supervision and formal teaching will increase your awareness of the evidence base of what you are doing in your workplace role. Teaching and learning alongside reflection on 'common sense knowledge' gained while on the job have the added benefit of providing objectivity to the process of learning because, as we all know, there are some things which seem to be common sense which are not! The use of WBL to enhance the quality of care you deliver supports a deep approach to learning which was discussed in Chapter 3.

The following Time Out activity gives you the opportunity to reflect on your own organization and your role within it.

Time Out: Considering your role within your organization

- **Can you identify your own organizational workforce plans?**
- **Do you know of any new emerging roles within your service?**
- **How could new roles contribute to the needs of your service?**
- **Are flexible courses, focused on WBL, available to support the needs of your organization?**
- **How does implementing new roles within your organization impact on your own future career development?**

Barriers to the adoption of WBL in the workplace

So far we have identified some of the potential organizational benefits of WBL. However, there are a number of reasons why an employer may choose not to adopt a WBL scheme in the workplace. These might include the financial cost, the nature of the WBL programme, not appreciating new ways of working, the poor press that some WBL programmes have attracted, the lack of flexibility within the competency element of some standardized WBL programmes in the past (such as **NVQs** and **SVQs**), poor inspection reports within the WBL sector (Smith 2003), the belief that there is not necessarily a relationship between working and learning (Beaney, 2004), and how busy the workplace is. Many universities and further education colleges will be happy to discuss the nature of the WBL programme with employers and adapt the programme to the specific needs of the organization, as we demonstrated earlier.

The lack of academic confidence in schemes of WBL is recognized by Walsh (2007), who feels that there is a need for the university sector to engage in gaining the confidence of employers in this type of provision, by adopting a new language of what she calls 'credit practice' which recognizes the virtues of both traditional and established academic working practices. Illeris (2003) argues, however, that the modern workplace needs to see beyond this scepticism, and recognize that adult learners are perhaps more inclined to learn when they can see the applicability of what they are learning to what it is they actually do in the workplace. There is also certainly the belief of the UK Learning and Skills Development Agency, who in a report into best practice in engaging employers in WBL state: 'Well-planned, on-the-job learning, with active employer involvement, leads to a better learning experience for learners and better outcomes in terms of their work-related skills and employability' (Taylor, 2001: 1).

As discussed earlier in Chapter 2, the culture that exists within the organization can create barriers to the adoption of WBL. Cultures that do not recognize the benefit of staff development will find it hard to keep pace with change and development within health and social care, so it is in the interests of organizations, even large ones like the NHS or Social Services, to adopt ways of working which promote this.

What this means for you as an individual employee looking to persuade your employer that WBL has things to offer the workplace, is that you will most certainly, in some instances, have your work cut out for you. Try the following Time Out activity to help you understand the barriers to WBL.

Time Out: Barriers to the adoption of WBL

Identify the barriers that exist to your learning in the workplace. These may include personal barriers such as lack of time and knowledge of how to go about this; team barriers such as work load and lack of motivation or organizational issues such as a culture that does not support WBL or a lack of belief in its benefits. Once you have made this list, you should spend some time reflecting on how you might overcome these barriers, what you will need to do, whose help you will need and how you might go about making a case for it. Don't forget it is imperative that you demonstrate that your plans for further learning are going to be of benefit to your employer and your organization and ultimately, and arguably most importantly, your clients.

Gaining your employer's support to undertake a Foundation Degree

So far we have looked at the benefits and challenges of adopting WBL within organizations, now we will turn our attention to why and how you might turn these to your own advantage. WBL may provide a great route for career progression for you because it provides you with the skills for work that fit the needs of your workplace, and as a consequence, makes you in turn more 'attractive' to your employer. Most employers will not want to invest either time or money in your training and development and then lose you to another organization!

For some individuals there are no established or traditional routes for self-development and you may need to spend some time identifying what the needs of your own organization are, as well as seeking out an appropriate course for you to help meet this need. The Time Out activities in this chapter will help you to do this but you should also refer to PDP in Chapter 7 and to guidance on developing career plans in Chapter 9. You should not be complacent about this because your appraiser may not have thought about your development or may not be aware of what is available to you. You may have to put the work in prior to your appraisal to identify the needs that your team or organization have, and what training is available to meet those needs. Currently, for example, there is an emphasis nationally on the development of Assistant Practitioner roles at

Band 4 with an FD qualification being largely required to fulfil this role. As the health-care sector works under increasing financial constraints to deliver high quality care for less money, future workforce development plans will place greater emphasis on this newly emerging specialist role. The work based element of the FD will ensure that you are fit for purpose and competent to undertake a Band 4 role as your learning and development would have been designed to meet your organization's needs.

So what arguments might you bring to the table when seeking support for your training and development? Certainly employers are looking for staff who have an awareness of the need for change and development, who are able to adapt to that change and embrace new and better ways of working. The skills that the course should offer should be flexible and transferable and bring added advantages to the workplace. Your employer will be looking for skills sets that enhance the likelihood of improving the organization's ability to survive and compete, and which enhance the image of the organization as one which provides top quality care. This sort of information can be found in the mission statement of any organization, an aware-ness of your organization's business plan and vision for the future will certainly help you identify a suitable WBL course, and make an argument for undertaking the training programme you identify.

Foundation Degree graduates' experiences of the benefits and challenges of WBL

Having emphasized the importance of understanding workplace culture, and obtaining employer and colleague support for further study, we felt it was important to share with you some past Foundation Degree graduates' experiences of studying a WBL programme. The following personal reflections demonstrate the joys and challenges associated with a Foundation Degree.

Personal reflections

Student 1

In this excerpt, a qualified Assistant Practitioner shares the experiences of undertaking an FD and relates what impact this has had on their career.

When I reflect on the FD, I call it my journey as I feel it has been like an epic voyage, which sounds very dramatic, although I can assure you, like life itself, this journey has had a lot of drama. I have felt the emotional lows of trying to understand lectures, work out what to write for assignments, missing time with family and friends or the frustration of not having enough faith in my own ability. The academic highs have been receiving notification that one by one I had passed the modules. The highs within my working environment have been through my newfound ability to work as a useful, confident team member, which has helped me develop into an Assistant Practitioner (AP) and, under the supervision of trained staff, am competent in helping provide

safe continuity of care to patients who come through the Department. Passing my Foundation Degree has been hard work and I am proud of my achievement. I feel as I did when I passed my driving test, I now have the underpinning knowledge and skills but my greatest challenges are to come, putting what I have learnt into practice, continuing to learn by guidance and experience and keeping my knowledge updated.

Within my workplace the FD has given me confidence in myself and my ability. I no longer walk past potential problems; I either deal with them or find someone that can. I look more closely at consenting issues and speak up when I need to. I understand the true meaning of respecting autonomy and am aware of different ways of communication. I am being asked for my opinions on improvement issues by those whom I asked for advice on my project. I find myself relating more and discussing issues with students on placement. Other care workers are asking me about the FD and I found myself enthusiastically selling it to them, although I explained emphatically I could not have achieved it without a good family support base.

Student 2

The student in the following example talks of the importance of seeking out support in meeting the educational challenges associated with undertaking a Foundation Degree.

The thought of attending university was a very daunting prospect. I was in awe of the place. It was a strange feeling being back in an educational environment, the last time was over 30 years ago. At first I felt out of place in campus with so many young students around, yes, I felt old, but soon blended in with everyone, and discovered it was a fun place to be.

The Foundation Degree Programme consisted of 12 modules, and I could only relate to three of them, namely the workplace practice modules. I did not know what to expect, so I attended those lectures with an open mind. I was not disappointed. At first there was some concern as to why we were studying these particular modules, the general feeling at the time was that they did not bear any significance to workplace practice. However, while attending the lectures I found that, yes, they did have some impact on workplace practice and in some instances of use in other modules. That was priceless. Evidence-based practice has made me a better practitioner and this was also achieved through searching and researching for information.

Pressure, stress, low morale, insecurity and personal concerns are just but a few barriers I encountered throughout the programme. However, each challenge was met and dealt with. The encouragement and support from tutors, other members within the group, colleagues from the workplace and family members achieved this. I could not have achieved this Foundation Degree without everyone's help.

These reflections demonstrate the importance of partnership working with workplace managers, mentors and colleagues in supporting a collaborative approach to not only your own individual learning, but to the organization as a whole. Undoubtedly, national evidence is starting to emerge that the Foundation Degree in Health and Social Care is fast becoming the recognized qualification for Assistant Practitioner roles which are part of a new flexible workforce for the future.

Chapter 9 provides you with an opportunity to explore your future career development in further detail integrating the main themes of this book.

Key learning points

- Organizations that place the importance of learning and development at the heart of their activities demonstrate the capacity to adapt to an ever changing health and social care context and are able to provide a supportive environment for WBL.

- We all have a responsibility to engage in lifelong learning to promote the quality of the evidence-based care we provide and the ongoing development of our workplace.

- WBL allows organizations to meet the needs of service users while developing their workforce.

- WBL can be tailored to the development needs of an organization in partnership with an academic institution such as a university or college.

- WBL helps to motive staff while on the job and to prepare them for future change and development.

- WBL allows the development of knowledge and skills by applying learning from experience embedded in practice.

- WBL offers a route to future career development and is especially useful in supporting the emergence of new roles in practice.

- Some organizations may not engage with WBL as they may not appreciate the relationship between working and learning and lack confidence in the awarding of academic recognition to this type of learning.

Critical review questions

- Can you identify three reasons why organizations might be sceptical about WBL?
- Can you list more than three examples of how WBL might benefit the working life of a health and social care organization?
- Can you prepare a good argument as to why your employer might allow you to take a course which is based on WBL, taking into account the benefits to them, to you and to your service users?

Web links and resources

Higher education academy on work based learning.
http://www.heacademy.ac.uk/assets/York/documents/ourwork/research/wbl_illuminating.pdf

Organizational cultures.
http://www.thetimes100.co.uk/theory/theory—corporate-organizational-culture—322.php

http://www.learnmanagement2.com/culture.htm

Lifelong Learning UK.
http://www.lluk.org/2788.htm

Business balls, a lighthearted and informative look at careers, business and training with a managerial twist.
http://www.businessballs.com/

References

Beaney, P. (2004) Founded on work? Work-based learning and Foundation Degrees, *Foundation Degree Forward*, 2: 8–10.

Clouder, L. (2009) 'Being responsible': students' perspectives on trust, risk and work-based learning, *Teaching in Higher Education*, 14(3): 289–301.

Geertz, C. (1973) *The Interpretation of Cultures: Selected Essays*. New York: Basic Books.

Herzberg, F. (1968) One more time: how do you motivate employees?, *Harvard Business Review*, 46(1): 53–62.

Higher Education Academy (2006) *Work-Based Learning: Illuminating the Higher Education Landscape*, York: The Higher Education Academy.

Illeris, K. (2003) Workplace learning and learning theory, *The Journal of Workplace Learning*, 15(4): 167–78.

Seden, J. (2003) Managers and their organizations, in J. Henderson and D. Atkinson (eds) *Managing Care in Context*. London: Routledge.

Smith, V. (2003) Raising retention and achievement in work-based learning, *Education and Training*, 45(5): 273–79.

Taylor, S. (2001) *Getting Employers Involved: Improving Work-Based Learning through Employer Links: Report and Good Practice Guidelines*. London: Learning and Skills Development Agency.

Walsh, A. (2007) Engendering debate: credit recognition of project-based workplace research, *The Journal of Workplace Learning*, 19(8): 497–510.

9 Career planning for the future

Where to from here?

Carolyn Jackson

Introduction

In the preceding chapters we reviewed the importance of work based learning (WBL) in the current health and social care context, outlining from a theoretical perspective why it has become important as a priority for the future, and from a practical perspective the sorts of knowledge, skills and attitudes you will need to develop if you are to be successful in your studies. In this final chapter, we explore some further tips and tools that will enable you to develop goals to plan your future career so that your activity is self-directed, you remain motivated and able to achieve what you want. Career planning is a lifetime process – you are always learning and growing, and as you do, your interests and needs also change. Career planning is not just about goal setting and making plans to obtain the career you want, it also helps you to make adjustments along the way because as we have seen, we learn throughout our lives. Most importantly good career planning enables you to find your passion in life and your joy in work, as well as identifying your place in this world, and fulfilling your destiny.

Upon completion of this chapter, you should be able to do the following:

1 Identify the benefits of career planning.

2 Use a range of tools to help you to identify the values, life events, personal and professional decisions that have impacted on your career plan to date.

3 Revisit and strengthen your personal development plan and career goals for the future.

4 Draw upon the findings from career coaching, annual appraisal, PDP and education and development opportunities to help you map your career timeline and plans for the future.

5 Use the NHS **Career Framework** and Skills for Health tools to help you to plan your career pathway for the next 2–5 years.

What are the benefits of having a career plan?

You need to plan your career because:

- planning assists in your development;

- you don't often stumble into your dream job;

- planning gives you a sense of accomplishment, especially when you complete things on your plan and begin to see personal and career growth; and

- you need to take personal responsibility for your own growth, no one else has a stronger interest in it than you.

The other benefits of having a career plan are that it enables you to develop particular skills and interests in your current post which add variety to your work and make you more effective in your role. It also helps you to develop specialized knowledge and skills in a particular clinical area or aspect of management, research or education. A career plan enables you to think about your future career to improve your capacity for promotion, or for making a career change. Finally it also enables you to achieve a more satisfying work–life balance to cope with life's challenges such as having young children, caring for elderly relatives, or coping with financial pressures.

Understanding yourself and what drives you

If you are going to make the most of your career plan for the future you need to make sure you understand yourself and what drives you. This book has already looked at a wide range of reflection skills, learning styles and tools to assist with personal development planning. All of these should have helped you to discover:

- your personal strengths;

- your career and job preferences;

- your motivation and priorities in life;

- how you want to balance your time between work and leisure;

- how you want to balance time and effort spent on work and income;

- what levels of responsibility, challenge and interaction with other people suit your personal style.

Take a little time now to revisit the activities you have undertaken in Chapters 3–7 and check that you understand what is important to you in your future career. You might like to review the SWOT analysis you undertook in Chapter 7 when developing your PDP, or indeed have another go here at analysing your current job role. This will help you to undertake a detailed look at your skills and strengths and where you are in your career at present. You can work through it on your own or with the help of a workplace mentor or group of colleagues. The aim is to help you note down as many of the strengths, weaknesses/challenges, opportunities and threats in relation to your current role as you can.

The following list summarizes some of the areas you might like to focus upon:

- *Strengths* and *weaknesses* of your role – relate to your knowledge, skills, experience, expertise, decision-making, communication skills, interprofessional relationships, time-keeping, organizational or practical skills.

- *Opportunities* – your experience in previous employment, or potential strengths you feel you have which includes transferable skills.

- *Threats* may include factors and circumstances that prevent you from achieving your aims for personal, professional or career development goals or service improvements. You can use the questions in Figure 9.1 to help you.

Strengths
- What do you do well?
- Why did you decide to take up the role you are currently working in?
- What makes you successful in your role?
- What knowledge, skills and expertise do you bring to your area of practice?

Weaknesses
- What are the common challenges you experience in the workplace?
- What skills could you improve on?
- Do you need to learn a new skill?

Opportunities
- What opportunities are there for you to undertake education and training add to your development that might create chances to develop your career?
- Are there any changes happening in the workplace at the moment that could help you to develop, e.g. a change in patient needs, new ways of working, new service improvements or strategies to enhance the quality of the service?
- Is there an opportunity to develop your career, e.g. through nurse training, continuing professional development courses, in house study days?

Threats
- What development obstacles do you face?
- Are the requirements for you to undertake your role successfully changing e.g. are you expected to have more qualifications to undertake your role?
- How do other people in your practice team feel about your role?
- Does the service plan to change its organisational structure and processes/procedures? If so what impact will this have on the skill mix of the team you work in and your role directly?

Figure 9.1 SWOT analysis of your career
Source: Chambers (2005).

Alternatively, another way of thinking about your future career is to undertake an exercise to help you to reflect upon and understand the career decisions you have made to date and ask yourself the question 'How did I get to where I am today?' A life timeline review exercise (Figure 9.2) is a useful tool to help you reflect on the highs

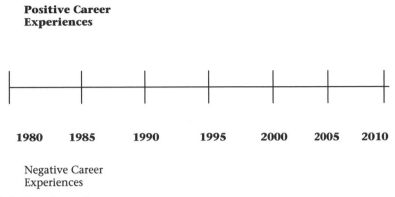

Figure 9.2 Timeline of your career

and lows of your career and enables you to look back at how your career path has worked out. You can learn a great deal about your relative strengths and weaknesses in this way. The idea is to plot career events and decisions you have made along the timeline and use the following reflective Time Out activity to help you structure your reflection.

Time Out: Reflection on Career

Ask yourself

- **If your career has been in a rut at periods in your past, what can you do now to take up the career opportunities available and optimize developments for yourself?**
- **Why do you think you can develop your career now if you have not done so in the past?**

Once you have completed this exercise you should explore the following questions:

- Is there a pattern to the line?

- What do the turning points have in common?

- What sort of events were crises for you?

It is helpful to try to take out a few examples and explore each in-depth. The following questions might help you to analyse your experiences further. You might also choose to undertake a SWOT analysis on each example you have identified to help with your analysis using the tools in Figure 9.1.

- What were your circumstances at the time?

- What were the factors that prevented you from developing your skills or progressing your career then?

- What were the factors at the time that encouraged you or enabled you to develop your career then?

To enable you to learn more from the timeline exercise try and answer the following questions:

- What does the timeline tell you about your attitude to taking risks in your career?

- Who do you believe are the people who have most influenced your career to date and why is that so?

- How do you think you have managed change in your career to date?

- If you were to extend the line to 2015, what would you hope the line would look like?

How do you develop your career plan?

Having reviewed your career history to the present day, it is important to consider what options exist for you to develop your career in the future. This is where a career action plan is helpful. It is important that your career action plan takes account of how you have behaved in the past and coped with both risk and change, and why you have perhaps changed (e.g. what personal life and professional circumstances have caused you to change). Think about what you want to do and find out what is required to help you get there.

One of the first stumbling blocks you might come across is trying to decide what options are open to you in planning your career. There are a number of useful tools you can use to help you as follows:

1 Use the opportunity to *undertake a short secondment* to a practice area that you are interested in working within in the future. This will enable you to demonstrate your transferable skills, help you to gain insight into the working practices of the service and ensure that you are making the right decision for a career move.

2 *Shadow a workplace colleague.* The purpose of shadowing assignments are to provide you with exposure to people who work in particular fields and to give you the opportunity to watch them in their day-to-day setting. Shadowing differs from secondment, because in a shadowing assignment, you are not there to do actual work, you are there to watch the other person do work. Shadowing offers the following benefits:

- the opportunity to watch someone 'in action';

- the opportunity to ask questions of someone while they are actually doing work;

- the opportunity to check out some of your assumptions about that particular field of work.

Shadowing is very much what the name implies, you follow the person around and watch what they do and what their day is like. Often they may get you involved in the task at hand, but the idea is not to do one type of work while they do another type somewhere else. This is your opportunity to be a sponge and watch what happens. The intent is to let you see what a day in the life of someone working in this field is like.

3 *Undertake an informational interview*. An informational interview involves interviewing someone about different jobs/career fields. The trick is to find someone to interview who will tell you what things are really like:

- What are the good parts of doing this particular job for a living?

- What are the bad parts?

- Do they really enjoy what they do?

- What's needed to get into this field?

Sources for informational interviews vary. It could be a workplace colleague who is working in that field, someone in personnel who can tell you what skills are required for that field, a manager or mentor who has people working for them in that field, or a combination of the above. These personnel can be great sources of information and take very little time and resources to conduct. The important thing is that you can use an interview to find out some really key information that will help your own career planning and decision-making such as:

- Tell me about your career progression.

- What is the most critical aspect of your job? Why?

- Did early career planning prepare you for your current job? If not, what did?

- How would you have prepared yourself differently?

- What type of career preparation would you recommend to someone who is aspiring to a career such as yours?

- What was your greatest career risk? Was this a successful experience?

- Have you used a mentor in the past or currently to help you identify areas for career development?

- What are your recommendations on how to enhance my opportunity to create a career in this field?

- What types of behavioural characteristics must one possess to be a successful _____?

4 Another great source of careers information is *websites*. Try the NHS Careers website http://www.nhscareers.nhs.uk/. The website provides access to a wide range of useful tools and resources that enable you to find out more about over 300 specific careers, the qualifications and experience required, and information about courses that will help you to develop your knowledge and skills further. It provides real-life stories of people who have done the job you are interested in and provides downloadable fact sheets to guide you. There is also an excellent web resource for Health Care Assistants provided by the Royal College of Nursing at http://www.rcn.org.uk/development/hca_toolkit.

The website provides a comprehensive toolkit that promote reflection and personal and professional development in the role for future career development planning.

Once you have tried one of these suggestions, you should be in a position to identify one or more career goals and understand the importance of being flexible about change so that you can take advantage of career opportunities as they come along. A career plan will also enable you to be proactive in adapting to the complexities of the health and social care workplace as it continues to go through a period of unpredictable change. With new Assistant Practitioner roles and responsibilities emerging at Band 4, and services being realigned for the future, it is important to know how these changes will impact on the service you work within, the roles that you occupy currently, and the effect this may have on your future career opportunities. Skills for Health, the Sector Skills Council for the UK health sector, aims to develop and manage national workforce competences and improve workforce skills. It has created a range of competences to describe what individuals need to do in their role and six national benchmark standards for Assistant Practitioner roles. Further information is available on their website: http://www.skillsforhealth.org.uk/.

Tips for managing lifelong learning throughout your career

We have seen throughout this book that the concept of lifelong learning (LLL) is central to enabling you to learn new skills, incorporate new knowledge, and develop new behaviours and attitudes throughout your life to keep pace with your life's changes. There are a number of key variables that support lifelong learning LLL:

1 *Understanding the influence of your workplace culture*. In Chapters 2 and 8 we explored the impact of workplace culture on learning in the workplace. Here we offer the opportunity for you to assess your current work culture so that you can understand the impact it has on your career development and progression. Try the Workplace Culture exercise in Figure 9.3.

2 *Personal Development Planning (PDP)*. Career development should be an integral part of your PDP which we explored in Chapter 7. Your PDP should set out goals for the forthcoming year and beyond, and describe realistic ways of achieving your career goals.

3 *Motivation*. You are more likely to want to progress your career if you feel motivated to do so. This comes from work that is seen as interesting or useful, where you are empowered to take responsibility, and have a sense of belonging and feel part of a team. This helps you to develop a sense of achievement through learning new skills or competencies in an environment where professional development is valued as an important aspect of career progression. It is really important that you take time and opportunity to find out what motivates and inspires you, and what does not. Your life experiences, your principles and values, your relationships with family, friends and colleagues, and work identity influence your career choices. The greater your self-awareness, the more satisfying your career choices could be.

Instructions: Read each number below then place a tick (√) in the appropriate Yes, Sometimes or No column that represents your experience.

Add the scores together at the end.
Yes responses = 2 points, Sometimes responses = 1 point, No responses = 0 points

My organization	Yes	Sometimes	No
1. Monitors the employee numbers on a regular basis to measure and track that we have the right number of employee ratios to the number of clients we provide a service for			
2. Monitors the turnover of employees on a regular basis to identify unusual peaks, trends and patterns that could result from internal or external factors			
3. Develops a plan for workforce development in advance for reasons such as promotion, retirements, turnover			
4. Makes appropriate investments in staff education, training and development initiatives to help employees build work-related competencies			
5. Invests resources in individual personal development plans for staff at all levels			
6. Provides adequate opportunities for career development that take into account managerial and supervisory needs			
7. Encourages staff to take accountability and responsibility for their individual learning and personal development so they will possess the necessary skills to be employable throughout their working lives			
8. Provides flexibility, facilities, services and programmes to support and enhance staff satisfaction and commitment to the organization			
9. Ensures that the expertise of staff knowledge and skills are matched to the right roles within the organization			
10. Provides career advice and counselling to staff			
11. Implements creative ways to reward and recognize staff achievements			
12. Creates a positive learning environment that encourages and supports staff involvement and engagement with core business and developments			

If the Score of your Organization was:	Then:
24-30 points	Congratulations! You are working in an environment that takes a flexible, positive approach to supporting its workforce and empowering them to take charge of their learning and development to meet future workforce needs and challenges.
15-23 points	More work needs to be done by the organization to support and develop its staff
14 points or below	Immediate work needs to begin on interacting with and developing staff in your organization. You can begin by modelling your own.

Figure 9.3 Self-assessment questionnaire about your organization's workplace culture

Source: Adapted from Rothwell et al. (2005).

Work values are very personal and vary from individual to individual. The sorts of things that motivate you at work can be classified into eight categories:

- technical or functional competence;

- general managerial competence;

- autonomy or independence;

- security or stability;

- entrepreneurial creativity;

- service or dedication to a cause;

- pure challenge;

- lifestyle.

You can define your work self-image in terms of these traits and develop a better understanding of your talents, motives and values – and which of these you would not give up if forced to make a choice. If you want to explore this further you can try an exercise on work values designed by the Royal College of Nursing at http://www.rcn.org.uk/__data/assets/pdf_file/0008/159515/Appraise_your_strengths_weaknesses_attributes_and_values.pdf.

4 *Making the most of your annual appraisal or performance review.* Your annual appraisal or performance review provides you with an opportunity to (i) reflect upon your achievements in the previous 12 months; (ii) to review your career action plan; (iii) identify further areas for growth and development; and (iv) to harness the support of your manager, multi-disciplinary team and workplace mentor in pursuing further training, education and development. It is a means to review career progression in terms of National Occupational Standards, Knowledge Skills Framework (KSFs) career progression bandings, your job and role description and explore opportunities to expand your role or learn new skills and competences. It should not be an annual paper exercise that is quickly completed and then put in a drawer for another 12 months. It should form part of a regular plan for your progression and development with your mentor and manager and should be reviewed every six months. The main purpose of annual appraisal is to do the following:

- Establish a common understanding between your manager (appraiser) and yourself (appraisee) regarding work expectations; mainly, the work to be accomplished and how that work is to be evaluated.

- Provide ongoing assessment of performance and the progress against work expectation. Provisions should be made for the regular feedback of information to clarify and modify the goals and expectations, to correct unacceptable performance before it was too late, and to reward superior performance with proper praise and recognition.

- Formally document performance through the completion of a performance and development appraisal form appropriate to the job.

- Construct a development plan for the coming year.

You should expect your manager to do the following:

- Translate organizational goals into your individual job objectives.

- Communicate their expectations regarding your performance.

- Provide feedback to you about your job performance in light of management's objectives.

- Coach you on how to achieve job objectives/requirements.

- Diagnose your strengths and weaknesses.

- Determine what kind of development activities might help you better utilize your skills to improve performance on the current job.

Ahead of your appraisal, read back over your SWOT analysis and Personal Development Plan for the year of appraisal. You might like to think about gathering the following information and feedback to help you to prepare:

- What are the good things about your job?

- What do you enjoy?

- In what areas do you think you are most skilled?

- What evidence do you have from your peers, mentor(s), workplace colleagues and clients that you are effective in your role?

- How can you maintain or improve those skills further?

- What are the things you enjoy least about your job?

- What could help to improve this?

- In what areas do you think you lack skills?

- How could you develop these skills for the future?

- What courses or training events have you attended over the past year?

- What courses or training events would you like to attend in the future?

5 *Working with a career mentor.* A career mentor is someone who has the time and ability to listen to you, and to help you in making decisions about your career. Some career mentors are only concerned with helping you to identify and meet your educational or training needs through a PDP, whereas others give practical or emotional support also. It is important to use the opportunity at annual appraisal to try and identify someone suitable who is prepared to work with you in this capacity. You should choose a career mentor wisely. They will normally be more experienced than you, and should have the knowledge and skills to be able to challenge you and prompt your career development. We would recommend that the mentoring meetings happen in work time for an hour every month or two. Using some of the tools to identify your skills, strengths and career plans included in this book will

help you to outline what you want to discuss with your mentor. It is important to use the opportunity to gain their perspective on how you have rated yourself and your career plans and to think about how career development features in your learning and development activities. You should share your current PDP with your mentor too.

Building a programme of educational study into your career plan

When thinking about the knowledge and skills you need to progress your career, you are likely to need to undertake some further training. As we mentioned earlier, the NHS Career Framework is a useful starting point for demonstrating how your post fits into the hierarchy of all NHS careers. You can also look on the Skills for Health website for a summary of the career framework and case study examples of job roles and their associated competencies. You can use this career tool to see what career options are available to you relating to your personal and practice commitments. http://www.skillsforhealth.org.uk/workforce-design-development/workforce-design-and-planning/tools-and-methodologies/career-frameworks.aspx.

If you are currently studying, or thinking about undertaking a Foundation Degree, you are likely to be employed as an Assistant Practitioner at Level 4 of the career framework. Assistant Practitioner roles are fairly new in the UK and there is a great deal of interest in the contribution they can make to the future quality of service provided by the NHS. Assistant Practitioners are involved in delivering protocol-based clinical care that was previously the remit of registered health professionals. This role is well established in some professions like radiography and has helped to develop a career structure for people who either want to advance, but do not wish to become registered health professionals, or for those who wish to gain professional qualifications. It gives the employer the opportunity to look at skill gaps within the team and decide at what level these should be filled.

An integral part of the development of this role is WBL through Foundation Degree study at Level 4 of the **National Qualifications Framework**. The FD is a higher education qualification worth 240 credits (similar to a Diploma in Higher Education) and usually takes between 2–3 years to complete. It gives learners a combination of technical, vocational, academic and transferable skills and is an important step on the skills escalator between NVQ Level 3 and full professional training. Graduates of an FD can expect undergraduate professional training to be reduced by one year.

There is an growing trend across NHS Trusts in England to employ Assistant Practitioners with an FD within defined scopes of practice. We share this with you as an example of new and exciting roles that are emerging in the modern health service. Here we present Paul's experience as a case study.

Case Study: Paul

Paul has recently qualified as an Assistant Theatre Practitioner. He started work in the NHS as a porter before taking the role of theatre support worker and prior to undertaking the Foundation Degree he had completed an NVQ Level 2. Although the trainee role represented an exciting challenge and was understood to be a workforce development, he was not at first fully aware of why the role was needed nor its potential impact.

He described the motivating influence of studying through work based learning and increased aspirations for his future career plan which was a significant personal achievement with his limited academic background.

His experiences are summarized as:

- the responsibility to raise awareness of the scope of the role within the department and increased ability to challenge practice issues;
- initial resistance from registered practitioners who were cautious about signing off competence due to responsibility and accountability issues. This mainly came from nurses rather than operating department practitioners;
- initial feelings of alienation and having to 'sell' the role himself;
- gaining improved understanding of the bigger picture within the department.

Some of the challenges he identified were:

- being considered neither a traditional student nor still a theatre support worker with loss of identity with his previous peer group;
- resolving issues around supervision with supervisors feeling they had to directly supervise at all times.

While the Association for Perioperative Practitioners supports the development of the support worker in the scrub role as contributing to the versatility of the perioperative team, thereby enhancing the role of the support worker, interpretation of the national guidance (Perioperative Care Collaborative 2007) initially challenged the value of the role within the theatre team. Interpretation of the standards and recommended practice led to the view that the requirement for direct supervision by a registered practitioner would require an additional member of the surgical team to be in theatre, thereby devaluing the role. A departmental policy detailing agreed operative procedures to be undertaken by support workers within robust clinical governance and risk management framework, ensured that the identified procedures and the delegated responsibilities were appropriate.

Continued professional development plans for qualified Assistant Practitioners within theatres include rotation between general, orthopaedic and gynaecological theatres to widen skills and create more workforce flexibility. The scope of

> practice is continually expanding within the service within an appropriate clinical governance framework to ensure appropriate management of risk. This includes ensuring that Assistant Practitioners are confident to decline undertaking a task if they are not competent.

This demonstrates the important partnership approach to work based learning between practitioner, workplace mentor and university course teachers in ensuring that a Foundation Degree prepares you for new and challenging roles in practice. It shows you that if you have the confidence and determination and support at work to undertake further study, it can make a real difference to your future career opportunities and preparation to fulfil new and exciting challenges.

This chapter has introduced you to the importance of creating a career plan for your future and given you tips for managing your lifelong learning.

Key learning points

1 Know yourself

- Review and update your CV on a regular basis as it provides a snapshot of your skills, expertise and experience at a glance.
- Reflect on what makes you tick, your leadership and decision-making styles, and the extent to which you are a team player.
- Be clear about what is important to you in your career.

2 Know what you want

- Know how much of a challenge you want in the future.
- Know how much you want to follow other people's guidance or lead.
- Know what kind of work–life balance suits you and how much financial income your want or need.

3 Know where you are

- Have a good understanding of your achievements and skills.
- Know your strengths and weaknesses.
- Understand your career anchors.

4 Know where you want to go

- Be aware of the options and opportunities open to you.
- Compare what is on offer with your responses to steps 1 and 2 above.

5 Know the gaps

- Analyse the gap between where you are now and the variety of options for where you want to be.

6 Know how to get there

- Have a range of strategies to bridge the gap in your career plan by using self-assessment toolkits, training, CPD and education opportunities.
- Develop a realistic action plan with contingencies for if, or when, your ideal career path does not work out.

7 Get support

- Find a strong career mentor for guidance and support.
- Develop a network of colleagues who are, or could, be important to you or informative about your future career. Try to extend this network beyond your everyday work colleagues to enrich your opportunity to share diverse experiences.

8 Know your workplace culture

- Find out what kind of workplace culture you work in. Knowing its strengths and limitations helps you to make decisions about your own career plan for the future.
- If the culture is impeding your development and holding you back, look for another culture or workplace that shares your workplace values and that invests resources in developing its staff.

Critical review questions

- Do you have a clear outline of what factors have influenced your career choices and decisions to date?
- Can you identify your skills, strengths and limitations within your current role?
- Do you have a career action plan in place with defined objectives for your future development?
- Are you planning to undertake a course of study to help you develop yourself further? If so, have you discussed this with your manager and course tutors?

Web links and resources

Provides valuable information about NHS careers and courses available to help you prepare for a wide variety of different roles.
www.nhscareers.nhs.uk

Provides a toolkit for health care assistants that links workplace job descriptions and roles to national standards and opportunities for interactive learning to achieve workplace competences.
http://www.rcn.org

Provides information regarding Assistant Practitioner standards.
www.skillsforhealth.org.uk

Reading for interest

Chambers, R. (2005) *Career Planning for Everyone in the NHS: The Toolkit.* Oxford: Radcliffe Publishing.

References

Chambers, R. (2005) *Career Planning for Everyone in the NHS: The Toolkit.* Oxford: Radcliffe Publishing.
Perioperative Care Collaborative (2007) Delegation: the Support Worker in the Scrub Role Perioperative Care Collaborative. PROPRIUS: London.
Rothwell, W., Jackson, R.D. and Knight, S. (2005) *Career Planning and Succession Management: Developing Your Organisation's Talent for Today and Tomorrow.* Westport, CT: Praeger.

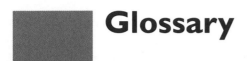

Glossary

Accreditation of prior experiential learning (APEL): the process by which academic credit can be awarded for the learning of knowledge and skills achieved by virtue of life experience and informal learning. APEL acknowledges that valuable learning occurs outside a formal educational setting and therefore is not formally assessed. Such learning can be achieved through workplace experience or outside work in a variety of settings. It is not experience itself that will earn academic credits, but the learning derived from reflecting on the experience.

Action learning: action learning is based upon the concept of learning by reflection (or reviewing) on an experience in which individuals, with support of colleagues, address problems, take actions to resolve those problems and learn from the process of doing so.

Action plan: a focused set of goals with defined activities in a set time frame.

Analytical writing: writing which is concise and to the point.

Career framework: provides a guide for NHS and partner organizations in implementing a flexible career. It enables an individual member of staff with transferable, competence-based skills to progress in a direction that meets workforce, service and individual needs.

Case study: involves an in-depth study of a single instance or event.

Clinical supervision: uses reflective practices and shared experiences to make sense of events in the workplace.

Common sense knowledge: the collection of everyday facts and information which we should all know.

Competency: the ability of an individual to undertake a defined task in a defined way to a set level. At the limits of competence the individual should be able to recognize when to ask for help.

Creativity: the ability to think through a subject or problem in new and inventive ways.

Critical incident analysis: an episode of our work that is significant and that we deem worthy of further scrutiny through reflection.

Critical incident record: the formal recording of a critical incident which aids learning through reflection.

Didactic: traditional approach to learning where the teacher instructs through the use of lectures with the student taking the passive role through listening, note taking, etc.

Empathetic writing: this is writing from a particular point of view which is sensitive to the client's current feelings and understood by the client.

Experiential learning: the process of making meaning from lived experiences.

Intellectual property: ownership rights of creative ideas which may be generated through work based learning activities.

Knowledge and Skills Framework: identifies the knowledge and skills that individuals in the health sector need to apply in their post.

Learning contract: a formal framework for structuring learning activities.

Learning cultures: cultures in which there is a willingness to adapt to change and learn new things in order to improve.

Learning diary: allows regular reflection on experiences allowing recognition of learning.

Learning environment: maximizes opportunities for formal and informal learning.

Learning organization: an organization which develops its staff so that it can meet changing needs.

Learning outcome: statement of a learning achievement.

Learning style: an individual's preferred learning approach and techniques

Mentor: a more experienced person who advises and acts as a guide for those who are developing.

National Occupational Standards: standards that describe competent performance in terms of outcomes. They allow a clear assessment of competence against nationally agreed standards of performance.

National Qualifications Framework: sets out the levels against which a qualification can be recognized in England, Wales and Northern Ireland.

National Vocational Qualifications (NVQs): work-based, practical qualifications acknowledged by employers and universities in the United Kingdom. They are awarded when people have proved their skills and understanding of various aspects of their work role. They are deemed to demonstrate that an individual is competent in their job.

Operational: the day-to-day running of the organization.

Organizational culture: refers to the values, beliefs and customs which exist in an organization. One example of organizational culture is the way in which the organization chooses to invest in the education of its employees.

Problem solving: an approach whereby the student is faced with a problem within the workplace where the exploration of ways to overcome the problem acts as a stimulus for learning.

Quality Assurance Agency: reviews the quality and standards of higher education in universities and colleges.

Reflection: consideration of experiences which allow alternative approaches to be considered.

Reflective diary/journal: a record of what has been learnt.

Reflective writing: making sense of an event.

Reflexivity: Being aware in the moment of what is influencing our internal and external response.

Scottish Vocational Qualifications (SVQs): work-based, practical qualifications acknowledged by employers and universities in Scotland. They are awarded when people have proved their skills and understanding of various aspects of their work role. They are deemed to demonstrate that an individual is competent in their job.

Strategic: long-term planning for an organization.

Tacit knowledge: knowledge that is gained through informal learning, i.e. in the workplace, which cannot be taught in the normal sense or rendered explicit.

Transferable skills: general skills which can be used in many jobs.

Tripartite: three-way; as in tripartite agreement between a learner, their employer and the education provider.

VARK: Visual, Auditory, Reading/writing, Kinaesthetic learning style.

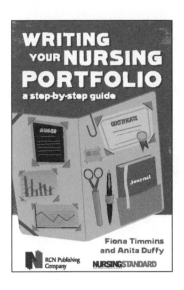

WRITING YOUR NURSING PORTFOLIO
A Step-by-step Guide

Fiona Timmins and Anita Duffy

9780335242849 (Paperback)
April 2011

eBook also available

This book is perfect for nurses who need to do a portfolio and don't know where to start. It explains simply what a portfolio can and cannot include, gives examples of good and bad pieces and demystifies the portfolio for the busy nurse. This is an essential purchase for qualified nurses doing PREP, and those studying who need a portfolio for assessment.

Key features:

- Provides suggested activities and tasks that can be completed and put into a portfolio
- Written as a 'step by step' guide
- Answers all the common questions nurses have about writing their portfolio

www.openup.co.uk

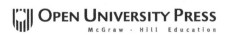 **OPEN UNIVERSITY PRESS**
McGraw · Hill Education

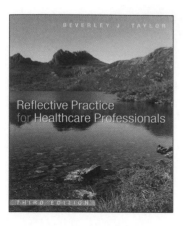

REFLECTIVE PRACTICE FOR HEALTHCARE PROFESSIONALS
Third Edition

Beverley J. Taylor

9780335238354 (Paperback)
2010

eBook also available

This popular book provides practical guidance for healthcare professionals wishing to reflect on their work and improve the way they undertake clinical procedures, interact with other people at work and deal with power issues. The new edition has been broadened in focus from nurses and midwives exclusively, to include all healthcare professionals.

Key features:

- Identifies the fundamentals of reflective practice and how and why it is embraced in healthcare professions
- Includes strategies for effective reflection
- Provides a step-by-step guide to applying the Taylor REFLECT model

www.openup.co.uk

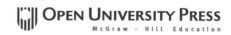

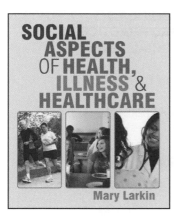

SOCIAL ASPECTS OF HEALTH, ILLNESS AND HEALTHCARE

Mary Larkin

9780335236626 (Paperback)
February 2011

eBook also available

This core textbook is the ideal companion text for health students studying social aspects of health and illness, whether it is part of a health studies degree or for a nursing or other professional qualification. Written at introductory level this is key reading for health students coming to the subject for the first time and looking for a broad and practical text.

Key features:

- Provides clear explanations of key concepts, extracts from primary sources, case studies and activities for study
- Explores and explains the different relationships between social categories and health
- Examines the role of the healthcare provider in society

www.openup.co.uk

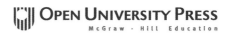

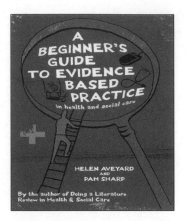

A BEGINNER'S GUIDE TO EVIDENCE-BASED PRACTICE IN HEALTH AND SOCIAL CARE

Helen Aveyard and Pam Sharp

9780335236039 (Paperback)
2009

eBook also available

This is **the** book for anyone who has ever wondered what evidence based practice is or how to relate it to practice. This accessible book presents the topic in a simple, easy to understand way, enabling those unfamiliar with evidence based practice to apply the concept to their practice and learning.

Key features:

- Provides an easy to follow guide to searching for evidence
- Explores how evidence can be applied in the practice setting
- Outlines how evidence can be incorporated into academic writing

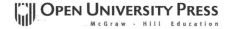

www.openup.co.uk